What People Are Saying About *But I Don't* Feel *Too Old* *to Be a Mommy!*

"This book for mature mothers and mothers-to-be gives a clear picture of what it means to have or adopt a child in your late thirties or well into your forties. Through the voices of real women and experts alike, Doreen Nagle's honest, comprehensive book tells the whole story. She gives you the courage to follow through with your dreams of motherhood—no matter what your age—and gives you every imaginable option for making them happen."

—Jennifer Hawthorne
coauthor, *Chicken Soup for the Mother's Soul* and
Chicken Soup for the Woman's Soul

"Finally a book that covers every aspect of becoming a mother beyond thirty-five and forty—from what to consider, to adoption, fertility and surrogacy options, to what the reality of everyday motherhood is like. Written with humor and frankness, the reader is hand-held every step of the way."

—Jeanine Cox
editor, *BabyZone.com*

"But I Don't Feel Too Old to Be a Mommy!" takes the worry out of becoming an older mother. It's the *'What to Expect'* for middle-life mothers."

—**Elizabeth Oakes,** forty-three
mother of two boys (six and three)

". . . phenomenal resource."

—**Mary Beth Sommons**
Chicago Tribune

But I Don't *Feel* Too Old to Be a Mommy!

The Complete Sourcebook for Starting (and Restarting) Motherhood Beyond 35 and After 40

Doreen Nagle

Health Communications, Inc.
Deerfield Beach, Florida

www.hci-online.com

Library of Congress Cataloging-in-Publication Data

Nagle, Doreen.
    But I don't feel too old to be a mommy! : the complete sourcebook for
starting (and restarting) motherhood beyond 35 and after 40 / Doreen Nagle.
    p.   cm.
    Includes bibliographical references.
    ISBN 1-55874-828-8 (tradepaper)
    1. Middle-aged mothers. 2. Older parents. 3. Motherhood. I. Title.

HQ759.43 .N34 2001
306.874'3—dc21

                        2001039230

Publisher: Health Communications, Inc.
              3201 S.W. 15th Street
              Deerfield Beach, FL 33442-8190

Cover design by Larissa Hise Henoch
Inside book design by Lawna Patterson Oldfield

For Hannah
from the Bronx

Contents

Part Three: Getting to Mommyhood

Foreword

As a little girl, my biggest dream was to be a mother. I courted fantasies of the extraordinary life my future children and I would share. Throughout my twenties and thirties, those imaginary little souls danced in my heart and floated in and out of my thoughts. Approaching forty and still single, I began to worry, would motherhood pass me by?

I got married when I was forty, and at forty-three was lucky enough to give birth to a beautiful baby girl. But I wondered: Is becoming a mother at forty-three any different than at twenty-three?

Motherhood past thirty-five and forty is an opportunity to make all those years of life experience work to your advantage. The path to midlife motherhood seldom runs in a straight line. Is it tougher to get pregnant as you get older? For many it is. Infertility may cause you to stumble, but it needn't block the path to creating a family; there's adoption or surrogacy as well as step- or foster-mothering. Likewise, today's older single woman who wants to become a mother also has many options. The door is open wider than ever before.

When it comes to midlife motherhood, overcoming obstacles is just par for the course. Most midlife moms discover they have infinitely more wisdom and patience than younger moms. Will you feel more tired than if you were younger? Likely, but think about it. Keeping up with your child forces you to take better care of yourself. There is no stronger motivation to eat healthy and exercise than the fear of having a two-year-old leave you panting in the sandbox.

In *But I Don't Feel Too Old to Be a Mommy!* Doreen Nagle intimately tells her own story and explains the special bond shared by women over thirty-five and forty who were not afraid to let their inner voice lead them to motherhood. She unravels the process and emotional issues involved in coming to motherhood later on.

The women in Doreen's book speak with a common voice. The motivation to become a mother at this particular time of their lives is always fueled by a powerful desire to raise and care for a child. I was especially touched by one adoptive mother's revelation. After four years of infertility treatment, she writes, "Yes, I was disappointed that I couldn't get pregnant. But the bottom line was that I wanted to become a mother, not a baby producer."

Nothing prepared me for the love I feel as I gaze upon my sleeping daughter's face. I can't fathom my life without her. Caring for her each day keeps the rest of my life in balance. Is being an older mother more challenging? Definitely. Do I ever wish I gave birth when I was younger? Sometimes. Do I ever regret my decision to have a baby in my forties? Never.

A year after Rebecca was born, I created an online midlife motherhood community as my solution to the feeling of isolation that sank in as a new baby turned my life upside down. *Midlifemommies.com* provides a forum for new older moms to share stories and gain support. I hope to see you there soon.

Rita Kennen
editor, *Midlife Mommies* (*www.midlifemommies.com*)
Mother to eight-year-old Rebecca

Acknowledgments

First, I wish to thank the many moms beyond thirty-five and over forty who shared their "been there, done that" experiences with me. You are the real stars of this book.

The highly respected fertility specialist, Dr. Eldon Schriock, gave his invaluable input and knowledgeable perspective on the fertility chapter and I am eternally grateful. Also, the well-known obstetrician, Dr. Hermina Salvador for giving of her time to read over the chapter on pregnancy and childbirth. Dr. Scott Coltrane shared intriguing research on family life.

I am most grateful to Carolyn Grayson, my literary agent, for believing in this book. Likewise to the gang at HCI, most especially Christine Belleris, my editor: Thanks for your ideas, enthusiasm and great wit.

Above all, thank you to my husband, Jules, who gave me the space and the place to write with his natural calm support—and to our son, Skyler, my inspiration. Life began when you showed up.

Who knew?!

An Introduction: Let's Get Started!

This Book Is Written for an Incredible Generation of Women: Ours

Our generation has done many remarkable things. Used to making headlines, we've pioneered trends that became commonplace: Some of us are the first generation of women to work outside of the home solely because we wanted to, not because we needed to financially. We look and feel terrific: We not only work out and eat healthy, we act, think, look and dress "younger" than counterparts in generations before us. We don't think of ourselves as "old." We're more confident than past generations in what we can accomplish at our ages. We are living lifestyles our mothers couldn't—or wouldn't—let themselves dream of.

No less a prestigious publication than *Atlantic Monthly*, in an article on assisted reproductive technologies (ART), referred to us as a "tough, feisty, indomitable group of women who are redefining what it means to age in the most profound way: by having babies who will enter kindergarten after their mothers celebrated their fiftieth birthday!"

Because we are pioneers, staring into the face of menopause as we simultaneously change our own kids' diapers doesn't seem so formidable to us. It's almost as if becoming mothers—commonly beyond thirty-five, increasingly after forty, not unheard of even beyond fifty!—is our natural next phase. We have instituted yet another societal change.

Even the experts know mothering later-in-life is not a flash-in-the-pan fad: "It's a phenomenon that's not going to change. Women delaying families is here to stay," declares Nanji Chandra, a demographer with the National Center for Health Statistics. A spokesperson for the National Center for Health Statistics concurs: "Even with more family-friendly workplaces, women will continue to become mothers over thirty-five in ever-growing numbers."

How Did We Get Here?

As the number of new or new-again mothers in the so-called traditional years (twenty to twenty-nine) declines, the number of new mothers over thirty-five continues to climb. A woman of forty just starting to think about forming a family is no longer an anomaly. Dr. Bernard Beck of Northwestern University agrees: "We will definitely see more older parents . . . It's a much more practical option today."

Right now more babies are born to women over forty than in the past four decades. (FYI: At the beginning of the 1900s, thirty-five and older was a traditional age for restarting motherhood.)

So, how did this happen? How *did* we get to be broaching midlife, baby lust in hand, while most of our friends are enjoying their grown children, spur-of-the-moment travel plans in hand? And how did some of us find ourselves playing with our grandkids with one hand and rocking our own baby's carriage with the other ?

"Life rarely happens according to the well-thought-out plans we made for ourselves when we were younger," one forty-three-year-old mother of twin five-year-olds told me. "Like a lot of other women I knew, I always thought I'd have kids, but I wanted all my ducks in a row first: a great income, a nice house. Oops."

Looking at it on the surface, the plethora of older mothers today makes sense: We as a generation haven't been very family-focused because, in part, we've been too busy. One new older mother sums up: "I was having a great life with a great job that I devoted a lot of time to. On the weekends we traveled, went to the theater, that sort of thing. Even though we had talked about wanting to start a family, it was always 'next year.' We were having so much fun time just flew by."

We are living longer and we are marrying later—not to mention more frequently. For some, the romantic notion that we'll meet Mr. Right, fall in love, marry and make babies either never happened or happened much later than we thought it might. Dr. Alex Steinleitner, a fertility specialist, says he and his wife met late in life and are trying to have a second child. "We're grappling with the same problems my patients are."

High divorce rates are another contributing factor.

Our generation is also at the forefront of making single motherhood an acceptable part of society. For those older mothers who are doing it alone, it took time to work their way through family and social prejudice; this in addition to the time it took to decide to try mothering as a single parent. By the time they decided to do it, many found themselves past the traditional years to start a family.

It's Definitely a Cultural Trend

"After making the necessary adjustments statistically, the number of older mothers is huge in comparison to the number of younger mothers, especially first-time mothers," said sociologist Dr. Scott Coltrane of the University of California, Riverside.

Another reason we delay motherhood is that we are a generation who works—whether strictly for pleasure or because there is a serious need. We've also been busy getting smart: more highly educated than our mothers, the National Center for Health Statistics reports first-time birth rates for women in their late late thirties to forties *with a degree* were two to five times the rate of women with less education. Over half of us are disproportionately well-educated and established in a career.

While not one trying-to-be or "already there" older mother I spoke with said they delayed motherhood in order to make a career their number-one priority—ambivalence takes that honor—we were very busy with our full lives. Babies never crossed our minds until we saw the pages of the calendar fly past us.

We Are Healthier . . .

Since we are in pretty good shape, age alone as an indicator of successful pregnancy is not the big factor it once was. As a matter of fact, age as the sole defining predictor of maternal health no longer exists. Our focus on caring for ourselves has forever changed the way forty-year-old women are perceived, especially by the medical community.

Desire Meets Technology

Not every reason we delay motherhood is by choice; some of us have tried for years to get pregnant without success. At last, the technology has caught up with our desires. If ever there was a time to be infertile, this apparently is it. It's also easier for the over-thirty-five crowd to adopt these days. As a matter of fact, it is so commonplace, an official with RESOLVE, a well-known adoption/infertility resource center, said it was virtually *un*common to find someone under thirty-five adopting today (generally, they are still trying to get pregnant).

Midlife Mothers Go Hollywood

In the celebrity community, becoming a mother beyond thirty-five and after forty has surpassed just plain trendiness: it's an everyday event. Yoko Ono made news when she became a mother over forty twenty-five years ago. Since then, the likes of Madonna, Vanna White, Jamie Lee Curtis, Camryn Manheim, Diane Keaton, Cheryl Tiegs, Rosie O'Donnell, Sally Field, Sharon Stone, Jane Seymour, Annette Bening, Bette Midler, Cybill Shepherd, Donna Mills, Connie Chung, Kelly Preston, Katey Sagal, Melissa Etheridge, Jane Kaczmarek and Adrienne Barbeau (she had twins at fifty-one with no fertility drugs!) have started (or restarted) motherhood later in life . . . and this is just a partial list.

This trend is not just the domain of the well-known. Look around your own neighborhood, workplace or park. It's likely you will come across a graying mom or two (or twenty!) with young kids.

Why This Book Was Written

Going through the process of trying to decide, then try-ing to become a later-in-life mommy myself, I found an appalling lack of information available to give me the sup-port, wisdom and insight that was necessary to choose the right thing for myself—and make me see that I wasn't: a) alone or b) crazy. For the most part, the books I found on the shelves dealt strictly with being thirty-five and preg-nant; but there is so much more to consider—from decid-ing to pursue the idea, to looking at options for motherhood beyond just pregnancy, to getting a glimpse of what parenthood is about. I also wanted to know what other women who had done it thought about it. Many of them were consulted in putting this book together—check out the Not-So-Secret Thoughts of Later-in-Life Moms chapter for their comments.

I learned a lot in researching this book; the vast majority of it is highly encouraging. One troubling fact that came up, however, is that women seem to be misled and/or ignorant of their fertility timeline. Many women think they'll get pregnant whenever they choose just because they feel they are ready to be a mother. This thinking severely underestimates the truth. *Seventy-five percent of women over thirty-five and forty experience fertility problems.* "The saying, 'It's never too late' was not meant for women who wait too long to get pregnant," shared obstetrical psychologist Dr. Roxanne Head.

Women who have not started families before thirty-five or forty have also been misled as to the numerous joys of later-in-life motherhood.

It is my hope this book will present for you a realistic and *complete* look at what to expect when you are "expecting to expect" a new child—especially when you are at a point in your life that you thought all this kind of stuff would be behind you.

As maturing women we are in a double bind: listening to the biological clock insistently ring can leave us yearning with midlife baby lust at a time when friends are becoming grandmothers. Should I? Shouldn't I? That's one of the questions I hope this book will help you answer. It is the intent of *But I Don't* Feel *Too Old to Be a Mommy!* to address the head, heart and facts of becoming a mother beyond thirty-five and after forty.

How the Book Works

But I Don't Feel *Too Old to Be a Mommy!* is written in four parts:

1. *In the Beginning:* Introduces the book, tells the author's story and shares some fun, as well as eye-opening, statistics.
2. *In Consideration of Mommyhood:* What to think about when choosing motherhood, the pros and cons, what the kids of later-in-life parents say, career options,

everyday parenting reality, special mothering circumstances—in other words, this section explores whether motherhood is right for you.

3. *Getting to Mommyhood:* Fertility technologies, pregnancy advances, adoption options, surrogacy, foster mothering, stepmothering, and single and lesbian mothering.

4. *Life Goes On:* Taking care of yourself beyond the beginning; Not-So-Secret Thoughts of Other Later-in-life Moms; Resources.

For Whom This Book Is Written

This book is written for those of you who are trying to decide whether you should go for it, as well as those who are in the process of doing it. It's also for those who have done it, and those who, along with their partners, friends and family, are just plain curious.

I kept all of you in mind as I wrote this book.

P.S.: About Being Labeled an "Older Mother"

The traditional years women start childrearing are twenty to twenty-nine; anything over that age has come to be known as "older," "later-in-life," "delayed" or "midlife" mothering. Let me say from the outset that I hate these limiting labels. Anyone in our age group considering motherhood knows we are anything but "old." With our looks, intelligence, creativity, spirit and wisdom, we certainly don't see ourselves that way and neither does anyone we know.

That's why I titled this book *But I Don't Feel Too Old to Be a Mommy!*

I've always believed that age is a state of mind; however true that might be, our bodies have been around longer than the bodies of women in the so-called traditional years. I like to think that we are older than they are in body only.

So, in lieu of calling us anything more original than these labels, it is with a sad heart that I feel forced to refer to women over thirty-five and forty as "older," "later-in-life" and (ever so occasionally) "midlife" throughout this book.

It is certainly not how I see any of you.

I invite you to help rectify this situation by creating a new word to describe our fabulous selves.

Then pass it on so that we may all benefit from its use.

PART ONE

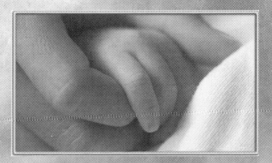

In the Beginning

CHAPTER 1

My Not-So-Unusual-and-Therefore-Worth-Telling Story

Nearing the end of our discussion for this book, I asked the highly regarded fertility specialist, Dr. Eldon Schriock, my standard final interview question: Was there anything else he felt we needed to address? I assumed he knew I meant in regard to the technical aspects of assisted reproductive technology, better known as ART.

"Yes!" he responded without hesitation, his up-to-that-point clinical nature nowhere to be found. *"Why do women wait so long to try to get pregnant?"* He was obviously frustrated.

My conversation with Schriock was just one of many opportunities I had been having lately to dissect, ponder and analyze that exact question: Most of my new friends were also later-in-life mothers. As a matter of fact, at the very first outing of our Moms Over Forty playgroup, the forty-four-year-old mother of twenty-month-old Trevor offhandedly asked why it took us all so long to "get here." I answered her with platitudes like, "Time flies." I wasn't meaning to be flip; I just didn't know how to explain, in twenty-five words or less, just what made me wait so long to start a family.

Truth be told, I couldn't point to a particular event or even a conscious thought that brought me to later-in-life motherhood. It was not anything I planned for. I couldn't remember one time when I ever, *ever* pictured myself pushing my first child's stroller while I was also pushing midlife.

It certainly wasn't how I envisioned my life turning out back when I was twenty, or even thirty; if I thought about family life at all, it was always to lay it off as next year's concern—maybe. Moreover, I wasn't the stereotypical "driven" career woman who needed three BMWs in the garage before there'd be a chubby-cheeked cherub in the "spare" room.

So how then, at an age when many of my contemporaries were taking time to stop and smell the roses, was I instead sniffing diapers? As these same contemporaries leisurely compared the color and texture of newfound wines, exotic vacations or newly decorated weekend cottages, my new mommy friends and I excitedly compared the color and texture of those diapers' contents, enjoying our discussions with as much gusto as our bacchanal-loving counterparts—maybe even more so!

Life Happens

The first day I held Skyler was my first wedding anniversary; but it certainly hadn't been my first wedding. As a young girl, I had a romantic vision that I'd marry and after a respectable, albeit brief, period of time, have children. I can even remember thinking that I'd "grow up" with my children, a thought put into my head by a friend who actually did start having kids right after an early marriage. I married my high school sweetheart, and we moved into Manhattan from our suburban lives. We lived the good life of Sunday champagne brunches; we both had fun jobs in publishing. If we wanted an exotic vacation, we took it. Times were too exciting to think of children. Frankly, I was too afraid of becoming a "housewife." My husband was adopted, and we always said that when (or if) the time came, we would follow suit. Trying to conceive was not an issue; trying *not* to conceive was.

Besides, we had cats. Did we really need kids?

Fast forward. It wasn't until my thirty-fifth birthday, when I was living in California, that I gave getting pregnant more than a passing thought. When I look back, I laugh at how obvious I was in responding to my biological clock. I would unconsciously rub my tummy and "feel" what it must be like to be pregnant. I would mime in front of the mirror arching my back forward into my stomach, even once bundling up a pillow under my shirt. I wanted to be pregnant; I'm not so sure I wanted to be a mother. The reality, while somewhat appealing, was quite scary.

I started some fertility treatments, but my husband's heart wasn't in it. Our hearts, apparently, were no longer in the marriage, either. After my divorce, it seemed that my longing for family life grew steadily. Was it because I was single for the first time in my adult life? Was it because my options were narrowing? Was it because it was a dream I thought I could never attain and therefore pined for?

Looking back, I think my desire came out of a real craving to have a more complete life; I had lived a pretty interesting lifestyle, stretching from the Big Apple to the Sierra to a boat on the San Francisco Bay, yet there was always a piece missing. The concept of becoming a mother started to take on a life of its own: I watched children more raptly, I envied my friends who had children (though most friends did not or had grown-up ones). Now, instead of eyeing single men, I would eye women with babies.

More than anything during that time, what weighed on me was the fact that I would probably always be childless since, for me, becoming a single mom seemed a road too long and too arduous to travel.

Then I met my present husband, Jules, the man who would become the father of our son. I immediately felt as if I had come home. In addition to falling in love again, one of the first things we talked about was a mutual desire for a family. He, too, was childless.

At this point, however, I was looking at forty from the far side and felt I didn't want to put my body through a pregnancy. To be honest, I was not aware of the advances in fertility that had been made in the few short years since I had gone through treatments. From hindsight, it is hard to know with certainty if I would have pursued assisted reproductive technologies even if I did know about the advances (I had very low progesterone so I knew I had problems). All I knew was that I didn't want to spend more time trying to get pregnant. I also didn't feel pressed to have a child only if it had my DNA; luckily, my new husband likewise didn't feel the need to become a daddy strictly through DNA. We immediately started looking into adoption.

Well, maybe not as immediately as we should have. Don't forget, after waiting as long as we both had to become parents, it was an overwhelming prospect. Would we be the oldest people in the PTA? We started meeting parents in our age group, happy graying mommies and daddies who showed us, just by being who they were, that we would not be an anomaly. Then we started the task of researching the finer points of adoption (see chapter 13) and chose a route to find our child—Russia!

From Russia, Came Love

Six months after we hired an adoption agency, we were in Kaliningrad, Russia. As we waited in the anteroom of the orphanage while they dressed our son that first day, I couldn't contain myself—we'd only seen video and photos of him thus far, not the real thing. Crazed with emotion, I screamed and cried as if possessed. I *was* possessed, possessed with a rapture I doubt I'll ever experience again.

At last, our beautiful son was handed to us. The first thing he did was touch my wedding band. Remember, it was our first wedding anniversary. One month later, Skyler turned one-year-old just two days before his father's birthday and one week before his mother's (a friend dubs it the Generic Family Birthday week).

Nothing will ever convince us that this child is not the one we were born to parent.

Shortly after we brought Skyler home, I was at story time with him. As the group of moms and kids sang and mimed "The Wheels on the Bus," I spied a woman about my age lurking in a corner watching us with envy. I remembered how I had felt before my gift from Russia, how I had longed to be "in the club." I smiled at the woman. She smiled back, and judging from her body shape and the size of her tummy, she wouldn't have long to wait before she'd be joining us with her little one.

CHAPTER 2

Statistics: The Good News, the Not So Good and the Just Plain Interesting

Here are some fascinating statistics about families and mommyhood:

- Three-quarters of divorced parents remarry, creating new stepfamilies.
- More than 40 percent of first marriages end in divorce.
- One in three Americans is also a stepparent, stepchild or stepsibling.
- Over one-quarter of families are stepfamilies.
- More than one million new stepfamilies are formed annually.
- A baby goes through about 350 disposable diapers in the first six weeks of life.

- Time spent in unpaid family work is equal to the time spent in paid labor (1997 study).

- Ten million mothers are running businesses out of their homes.

- Seventy percent of mothers who start a business at home leverage a former career into a home-based career.

- Two-thirds of women in the workforce are mothers.

- More than 60 percent of kids in first grade through high school have mothers who work at least part time outside of the house.

- Luxembourg's state-mandated leave provides up to ten weeks paid maternity leave. It is one of the *least* generous leaves in Europe. By comparison, the U.S. only allows for twelve weeks of *unpaid* leave and only for those women working in companies with over one hundred employees.

- Italy provides up to five months fully paid leave.

- In a 1998 Current Population Survey, in households where both a husband and wife lived, women were listed as head of household in 23 percent of the families.

- In total, one in five kids in the United States lives in a household headed by a mother.

- One out of every six dollars a single mother earns goes to childcare.

- In a poll, two-thirds of men and women agreed that income and housework should be shared equally.

- The greatest number (84 percent) of those who agreed with this (above) statement were unmarried.

- In 1992, 66.7 percent of women twenty to twenty-four were childless. In 1960, 47.5 percent were childless in that same age group.

- Twenty million families in the United States have only one child.

- The heart pumps 50 percent more blood when a woman is pregnant versus when she is not.

- Women have about four hundred menstrual cycles in a lifetime.

- Long menstrual cycles coupled with high levels of stress may result in infertility, reports *Family Practice News.*

- Three-quarters of all embryos end in miscarriage.

- Over 80 percent of women in the United States eventually become mothers.

- Mothers over forty give birth to more left-handed babies. Lefties are usually shorter and weigh less than righties. Presidents Reagan, Clinton and Bush Sr. were all lefties.

- In the last decade of the twentieth century, the number of professional women grew by 60 percent.

- The United States is the largest importer of internationally adopted children in the world.

- The majority of women who adopt are over thirty-five; most are over forty.

- The United States has the highest teen pregnancy rate of any developed country.

- Of all the children born to teenagers, only 3 percent are offered for adoption.

- Almost all mothers everywhere carry their babies on their left sides—where the heart is—whether or not they are left-handed.

- Only 5 percent of women delay motherhood because of a career.

- The current average student loan is fifteen thousand dollars.

- There have been about ten thousand surrogate births worldwide.

- A Beth Israel-Deaconess Medical Center study concluded that women who give birth later in life are slower to age.

- The average person today lives about thirty years past retirement.

- People work an average of 50 percent of their life span. That means 50 percent of their lifespan is *not* spent working.

- *The Journal of Nature* reports that nearly 20 percent of

women who live past one hundred gave birth after the age of forty.

- There was a 92 percent increase in the number of women giving birth over forty from 1980 to 1989.

- Ninety-seven percent of newborns do not have serious birth defects.

- The fertility business has grown to over $2.6 billion dollars, up $1 billion in just three years.

- A *Parents Magazine* survey shows couples are twice as likely to kiss their new child as each other.

- There are about 520,000 children aged newborn to eighteen in foster care. Of that number, 21,000 are under one.

- An estimated 117,000 children in foster care are available for adoption. Thirty-five percent are between ages one and five.

- The number of children in foster care has risen 89 percent since 1982.

- Urban areas have larger older-parent populations.

- First-time birth rates for women with degrees who are in their late thirties through their forties were two to five times the rate for women with less education.

- Seventy-five percent of women over forty who get pregnant do so only as a result of fertility treatments.

- Without fertility treatments, chances of pregnancy for

women under thirty is 20 percent in any one month; 5 percent for women forty and above.

- Births to women in their early forties have doubled in the last thirty years.
- Four million American women deliver babies each year.
- One in five pregnant women over forty gives birth to her first child.
- Only one in four obstetricians deliver fewer than ten babies a month.
- One-quarter of pregnant women do not see a doctor until after the twelfth week of pregnancy.
- At the turn of the last century, one in one hundred women died in childbirth. By the turn of this century, those numbers dropped to one in fifteen thousand.
- An online poll asked women who stresses them most:
    Boss: 14 percent
    Kids: 36 percent
    Husband: 50 percent
- Of the women who turned fifty in 1998, 17.5 percent had only one child. That is a 10 percent increase over the decade before.
- In 1800, there was an average of 7 children per family. In 1900 there were 3.5 per family. In 1990, that number had dwindled to 2 per family.
- Of those responding to a fall 2000 childcare survey:

70 percent say one parent should stay home full time.
14 percent believe parents should work different shifts.
6 percent want a close relative to be the caregiver.

• Of those who use day care, a babysitter at home or a
reliable neighbor for childcare, 62 percent say they are
very happy with their arrangements.

• Two to one, people who responded to a survey on
childcare said it should be made easier for one parent
to stay at home rather than improve the state of
childcare.

• 4.5 million children need childcare in the United States.

• Multiple births have increased in the last twenty-five
years mainly because of fertility drugs.

• Multiple-birth odds increase in direct proportion to
the age of the mother: older mothers are more likely to
have multiples even without the aid of fertility drugs.

• Eighty-five percent of miscarriages occur in the first
trimester.

• Mt. Sinai hospital found older mothers were no more
likely to have preterm, low-weight or stillborn babies if
they were generally healthy.

• Risk factors for pregnant women increase over thirty-
five as well as under twenty.

• The risk of fetal chromosomal abnormality is less than

1 percent in women over thirty-five; 3 percent in women forty-five.

- Premenopause starts around forty-five; menopause occurs generally between fifty and fifty-five.

- Sixty percent of the children born in the United States during the 1990s will spend a portion of their childhood fatherless.

- Oak trees do not produce acorns until they are fifty years old.

- As many as five people can be involved in an assisted reproductive technology (ART) birth: sperm donor, egg donor, gestational (a.k.a. birth) mother and contracting mother and father.

- The first baby born by in vitro fertilization was born in Cambridge, England, in 1978. Since then, more than 300,000 babies have been given life through IVF.

- The average baby born in the United States weighs seven pounds, seven ounces.

- By 1993, more than half a million U.S. children were born to mothers under twenty and another half-million born to mothers over thirty-five.

- According to the Work and Family Institute, three-quarters of all women with children under five will work for some of the time while their children are still in school.

PART TWO

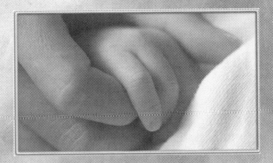

In Consideration
of Mommyhood

CHAPTER 3

The Pros and Cons

J ust about everything we do has an up side
and a down side. Delaying motherhood is
no exception.

There are lots of myths associated with
becoming a mother later in life; then there are
the realities. Let's get the not-so-good ones
out of the way first . . . then stay tuned for the
plentiful positive aspects of motherhood over
thirty-five and forty.

Disadvantages

Less Energy

It's the single biggest worry potential
mothers in this age group have: "Will I have

the energy to keep up with my child?" A decline in energy is a natural part of getting older; after all, we have more years under our belts than our younger counterparts. Motherhood or not, the mere reality of those years translates to more stress on our bodies and accompanying lowered levels of energy. But don't count older mothers out of the game just yet. First of all, as a group we take pretty good care of ourselves. Second, thirty-five and forty are no longer considered "old" by any stretch of the imagination. Mom versus mom, it's not a foregone conclusion that you will have less energy than the twenty-year-old moms in your playgroup. Glance around the next time you go to the park. Plenty of younger mothers look pretty pooped after chasing their toddlers while lots of older ones are energized doing the same thing.

Look on the bright side: As one over-forty mom of a sixteen-month-old explained, "It works out great. My son and I are on the same nap schedule."

The Need for Privacy

Privacy is important for *everyone*. The fear of loss of privacy is a big issue in any new living-together relationship, be it adult-and-adult or child-and-adult. Women who have waited to become mothers are most likely used to getting a lot of privacy if they've been childless, or if they have older children off doing their own thing.

Getting privacy when there are children in the house is manageable; it just requires some planning. For example, wait till nap time to get privacy for your bubble bath. As your child grows, more can be explained about your (and his or her) need for privacy. Boundaries can be more firmly drawn.

As long as your child is safe and occupied, it is not your responsibility to entertain him or her every waking moment.

OPQs and Cs

OPQs and Cs translates to Other People's Questions and Comments—the unwanted kind. Some people feel they have a right to say anything to you about your decision: "Is that baby *yours?!*" ("You bet! Just like these wrinkles.") "Aren't you too old?" ("Aren't you too nosey?") "Why would you want to change diapers at *your* age?" ("Were you offering to change them for me?") Television character Murphy Brown, upon announcing her pregnancy (at forty-three), was greeted with the rhetorical, "What is this? Some kind of premenopausal insanity?" Remarks like these often come from people who already have children and can't remember their own yearning to parent. While they might turn their noses up (literally) at the thought of dirty diapers, you're likely to be grateful for every piece of poop you find there.

You have choices: You could spend your time coming up with snappy answers to these very personal questions, educate people to the realities of your decision or ignore them. Regardless, realize that people are more than likely just curious about this relatively newish and growing (yet definitely *not* uncommon) phenomenon called delayed motherhood.

And it's not just strangers: Even so-called supportive friends and family members who ostensibly only want what makes you happy can get in on the act by asking, "Are you sure you know what you're doing?"

Maybe not. But do they always know what they're doing?

Work, Work, Work

Unless you are sitting in the catbird seat when it comes to money, you may wind up having to work at least part-time past the traditional retirement age in order to pay for your child's college and your own "senior citizen" needs.

Mothers who delayed motherhood won't be the only ones working into their later years. Word is our generation will be working well into their seventies, young children at home or not. Even those who can afford to retire won't, say the experts. Because we are living longer in healthier ways, we will want to continue to be active and engage in some style of work; many of us will have at least a small home-based business.

Older Moms, Older Dads: Same Old Double Standard

Clint Eastwood had his seventh child with his fifth wife when he was sixty-seven. Reports consistently praised him for "settling down." Tony Randall had his first child at age seventy-seven; a year and a half later he had his second, making him the media darling of that year.

Contrast this with the sixty-three-year-old woman who became the world's oldest mother to give birth. *She* had to hide herself and her family from the media because of negative reaction. Then there's the sixty-one-year-old British woman who had to fight for fertility treatments so she could have another baby after her only child had been killed at age eighteen. London fertility specialists turned her down because they thought she'd be too old to handle the stress of *motherhood*, not the stress of *pregnancy!*

Fertility specialists can't agree on how old is too old for a woman to bear a child. While some don't know whether they should ever say no to a woman wanting to get pregnant, most fertility programs will not work with women over fifty-five.

There are no age cutoffs for men.

Antiquated thinking prompts some doctors to show their prejudice: Dr. Arthur Caplan of the University of Minnesota says that children have a right to a mother who won't be entering a nursing home while they are heading to

high school. Apparently the doctor (and the fertility industry in general) does not find this argument relevant to dads.
Deeply entrenched prejudices against women becoming
older mothers exists partly out of the fear the child will be
left motherless at a young age. Why isn't there equal concern about older fathers leaving a young child fatherless?
Are we trying to say that only women make effective or
important parents? Don't daddies count?

Frustrated Italian fertility specialist Dr. Severino Antinori
views the disparity this way: "A man can have a baby in later
years and people say, 'Isn't he clever?' But those same people
say an older woman is a dishrag."

While criticism of women on the outreaches of "older"
mothering is not unusual, the tide seems to be turning. A
recent *Family Circle* magazine survey shows that over two-
thirds of their readers support fertility treatments for older
mothers. "If it helps women become mothers, it's a good
thing," the readers concluded. This attitude has progressed
from where it was even a few years ago.

A Loss of Generations

If you wait a long time to become a mother, your child
will likely not have the same extended family to grow up
with that his classmates with younger parents do. Great-
grandparents—and in many cases even grandparents—will
not be around for him or her.

Parents in their twenties have typically three or four generations of family members to offer their children; those in their forties typically have one or two (themselves and their own parents). "Many younger parents have their own youngish parents to count on if they need help or want to get away for the weekend without the kids. Our parents were in their late seventies when we finally had Hannah, so we couldn't count on them in the same ways," says one over-forty mother of three children, all under five.

You can fill in the gaps by putting together a strong extended family of friends for your child, which might require a lot of work. Also remind yourself that not all children have large, warm and loving "Norman Rockwell" families, no matter how old their mothers are.

Later Mothers Have a Tendency to Rush Their Infants to "Do Something"

Probably true. Many women who have waited to start or restart their families want to catch up on time "lost." They are often guilty of trying to push their infants to talk, walk or read sooner than they'd be ready to. One first-time mom is typical: "I'm so anxious to start doing all the things I've been dreaming I'd do with my own child—like riding bikes or going to the movies—and he doesn't even talk yet! I want him to hurry up and do things!"

Each stage is wonderful. Enjoy it.

Later Mothers Wrap Themselves Up Too Much in Their Children

Again, this can be true, especially of women who have given up interesting careers to be stay-at-home moms. These are women used to putting their full focus on their careers. Motherhood is now that career. This can turn into a problem when the mother becomes so enmeshed in the child's outcome (how smart, cute, likeable, athletic, etc. he or she is), rather than focusing on the love, fun and growing bond between them.

Are You Part of the "Sandwich Generation"?

Will you care for aging parents while at the same time mothering your own young children and saving for college tuition? Raising children and caring for aging parents are each intense, time-consuming and emotionally draining commitments leaving little free time for the mother/caregiver trapped in the middle. Luckily, today there is a depth of understanding of how hard this situation can be. As a result, a wealth of information and support exists, from books to organizations of kindred spirits offering good advice and more.

Finding Peers

No, it's not as easy to find mothers with young children in your age group in some areas. To find mothers in your own age group, check out resources in your community. These can include local parenting publications, childcare providers, adoption agencies, story time, church or synagogue, Mommy 'n' Me classes or the park on a sunny weekday morning.

Some communities are more likely to attract older mothers than others (e.g., metropolitan areas). If you can't find a group of women your age with young children, start one. (See Chapter 7, "Reality Bites," for specific how-to's.)

"But Aren't I Being Selfish to Have a Child at My Age?"

Probably. Nine out of ten reasons *anyone* has for wanting a child are selfish.

Even (Some of) Those Who Are Doing It Aren't So Sure They Should

I was surprised to find that even amongst women who are (or who are becoming) later-in-life mothers, there is controversy and sometimes embarrassment about their age. Feeling their situation was "too personal to share their stories, even anonymously," one can't help but wonder which came first: their own feelings or public perception?

The majority, however, were proud, thrilled and feeling privileged.

Advantages

These Children Are Advantaged

A 1993 university study found that mothers in this age group are not only more educated as a group, but they "bring a tremendous amount to a child. They have more life experience and therefore can impart more advantages to their children." Furthermore, these women were found to be grateful that they were able to become mothers after delaying motherhood and were very appreciative of their newfound role. As opposed to feeling resentful that they were now "tied down" to family life, these women felt that they were at last on the "inside track."

The study also found that older parents were better at talking to children like they are "real people."

On the flip side, many of these mothers were found to have unrealistic expectations of themselves. After years of having to be a "perfect" employee, they believe they have to be a "perfect" mother.

Ready for It

Few older mothers get pregnant by chance; no one ever adopted by accident. Women who delay motherhood have given it a lot of thought and often go through a lot to get their children—from arduous, expensive and often disappointing infertility treatments to sometimes humiliating adoption procedures. They are not merely appreciative of the gift of motherhood, they are chomping at the bit, rarin' to go in their new role! They've been there, done that—made decisions based solely on their own needs, spent their free time as they saw fit, did likewise with their money. Their emotional, spiritual and sometimes physical health are better than when they were in their twenties.

Another Way Older Women Are Ready

When an older mother says she would not have been as good a mother in her twenties as she is in her forties, she often means she wouldn't have been "able" to give her child the attention he or she needed. She may not have had enough life experience under her belt to have worked through her own development issues in her early twenties in order to center herself on a child as much as she did when older.

"If I had had children in my twenties, I would have been frozen with all the responsibility—decisions and things—the 'stuff' that needs to be attended to," a new mother age forty-three said.

When all is said and done, motherhood is more about being ready for it than the age of the mother.

Less Focus on Self

A surprising by-product of becoming a mother after so many years of being without little ones is that it forces you to stop being the center of your own universe; in other words, to stop being self-centered. Along with the responsibility of mothering comes limited time for indulgences into self-pity or trivial matters. You live a less outwardly focused life. Many women interviewed for this book said that if they had had a baby earlier on, their children would have lost the fight for who is the most important member of the family: Mom would have won hands down.

Patience

Who amongst us hasn't become more tolerant with every passing year? This spills over into mothering in big, important ways. Older mothers have a tendency to be more forgiving, talk things out with their children, brag rather than freak-out when their tiny ones start drawing on the wall. Patience is a requirement in raising an independent child.

Cautious But Not Overly Concerned

A kindred spirit to patience is lessened anxiety. When it comes to allowing their children to take calculated age-appropriate risks, many older mothers find themselves allowing—indeed, encouraging—their children. They often err on the side of cautious permissiveness because they are more relaxed.

This comes from more . . .

. . . Self-Confidence

As someone who brings the wisdom of maturity to mothering, the older mother is more confident in her abilities as a parent. She knows herself better and therefore can raise her child with a steadier hand. She'll also be more likely to fend off unwanted parenting advice and stick to her guns when friends insist she is doing it wrong. This works not only to her advantage, but to her child's benefit: The values she brings are well thought-out.

Humor

Skyler was about one-year-old when I found myself lugging a new microwave around the mall with us. It was past his nap time; he was sticky from the wrong kind of snacks. He refused to stay in the shopping cart seat, so I had to push the cart with my hip while holding onto him as he screamed—loudly—his rear end tossing between the handle and the seat. Our car was parked clear across the other end of the enormous parking lot, and it was raining. Hard.

Oh, and his diaper reeked.

The looks I got from passersby ranged from empathy to "Hey, lady! Can't you control your kid?" (Apparently not!)

I reacted like any new older mother in my shoes would have—with laughter, absolutely blessed to have this experience in my life.

I still find myself laughing in the midst of situations that I am pretty convinced would not be so humorous to me had I been younger. Indeed, I probably would have been one of the passersby clicking my tongue in disapproval. What a difference a few years make!

Don't Have Time to Play Anymore?

You will now. As a matter of fact, both your inner and outer child will be forced to play on a daily basis. Here's a chance to let loose, be goofy, make silly faces, utter ridiculous noises all to very favorable audience review—so go ahead and take advantage.

Money

Because many older mothers may have had more of a chance to establish a solid career prior to motherhood, they may be able to afford extras for their child while also maintaining those aspects of their old lifestyle that money can buy: nice clothes, additions to their homes, fun vacations. As a result, more solid finances are cited as one reason women delay motherhood in a study of children of older mothers.

Motivated Parenting

More findings from the aforementioned study: Mothers who are older dive into their new job with both feet. The study concluded, "They tend to put more energy into the job of being a parent." They are more likely to read about parenting and apply what they read as well as attend to their child's school years and family-oriented leisure in deeper ways. Putting off motherhood has given these women ample opportunity to study the parenting struggles and styles of others; they can pick and choose from those examples to see what works best.

As a result, kids of older parents are called "advantaged," since they have a lot of favorable attention paid to them by older parents who adore them.

Widening Social Circle and Experiences

Having kids is a great way to meet new people who have the same interests you have—the raising, loving and enjoyment of a child. You'll have ample opportunity to meet these people, aside from the obvious ways: oohing and ahhing over each other's little bundle of joy at the supermarket is one way you probably hadn't thought of.

You will also learn new things as you become privy to what goes on in tumbling class and how an intelligent woman can spend an hour discussing the merits of one kind of toy versus another with her new mommy friends.

Motherhood Keeps You Younger

It's a fact that keeping up with your child will keep you young mentally, but now there is proof that older mothers who give birth live longer: A Boston study says that women who have given birth after the age of forty may be four times more likely to outlive their non-childbirthing counterparts. The study concludes that later pregnancies are a sign that the reproductive system is aging more slowly, which could mean a later menopause: Estrogen loss, therefore, is delayed and can reduce the risk of heart disease and stroke.

The study warns, however, that you should not conclude that if you have difficulty conceiving past age forty, it signifies an early death.

Another study of sixty-nine couples says that older parents take better care of themselves, staying mentally young with more mental resiliency. Later mothers have more tendency to take care of themselves. "Having my child made me want to take a look at my lifestyle and eat better and exercise regularly. Every time I don't want to get on the treadmill, I think about how many more years I have to go keeping up with her, and I force myself off to the gym," a fit forty-four-year-old mother of a nine-month-old says.

Read chapter 15, "In It for the Long Haul," for more ways to care for yourself.

And Finally, for All Those People Who Waited . . .

Friends and family who waited for you to become a mother will be so happy that you have done it at last, that they'll offer to babysit so you can escape for a dinner out.

Well, at least once.

CHAPTER 4

Everything You Need to Make a Decision About Becoming a Later-in-Life Mommy . . . Except Someone to Make It for You

Your parents long ago gave up hinting that they want to become grandparents; ditto friends who insist "for your own good" that if you are going to have another child, you better "do it now." The alarm on your biological clock is about to explode and, considering the date on your birth certificate, even you can't explain why you have a sudden newfound urge to be a mommy.

No wonder friends and family are confused.

Perhaps your delay in growing a family hasn't been by choice; after all, you stopped using birth control a long time ago and thought you'd be pregnant by now. Or maybe you didn't find that perfect mate until you were in your thirties, and it's taken time to figure out whether you want to be parents or not.

Choosing motherhood later in life may appear to be a case of your heart overruling your head—while fantasies of the perfect family dance in your brain—but your head knows that time is of the essence.

The decision to become a mother should be thoughtful and personal. It requires soul-searching as well as peacemaking between your heart and head. No matter what you choose, it is a life-changing, lifelong decision; but don't let that scare you. Motherhood later in life *is* indeed life-changing—for the much, *much* better (excuse my prejudice for showing)!

If you've delayed motherhood thus far—or delayed restarting motherhood—beating yourself up with, "Why didn't I do this sooner?" will only create more regrets. Instead, take action. Delaying the decision any longer is fruitless.

In helping you think it through, you can—and most likely will—get all the advice you want, solicited or not. Choose wisely with whom you confer: Many well-intentioned friends will share their knowledge of later-in-life motherhood based on information twenty or more years old. Remember, too, when all is said and done, no one can guarantee motherhood *at any age* will run a smooth course.

The bottom line is this: You can explore the issues analytically all you want, but if the desire is deep within, it will propel you to follow it. "I know there are decisions where I have to act on my gut alone," one forty-year-old who is trying to conceive confessed. "Some things I just can't trust my head with."

This chapter was written to help you in your decision-making process: to give you food for thought so you can feed your soul—whether you are considering motherhood for the first time or all over again.

Ready or Not: The Big Three to Consider

1. How old is too old?

While options for getting to motherhood are not as open-ended as we get older (i.e., take fertility: It borders on non-existent for a woman in her late forties), they are by no means over with. "Two hundred years ago childbearing women were dead by thirty," says author Erica Jong in her book, *Fear of Fifty.* "Today, many of my friends are becoming mothers in their forties. We have extended the limits of life."

What seems old to one woman may seem like the start of springtime to another. How you feel physically, mentally, financially and culturally has much to do with it. Then there are the practical issues that need to be considered: Will your child be taking care of you just as he or she is starting out on his or her own? Should you set a time limit on trying to get pregnant or working toward adoption?

Some things can be worked out with pencil and paper. Other concerns are less tangible and rational. Take the top most oft-stated reason for delaying childrearing:

2. Fear of parenting

Middle-life women who teeter on the fence about mothering admit they are afraid of motherhood even as they crave it. Like anything else untried, images of what might be required of them grow in their heads. Will they be able to live up to the requirements? What if they do it "wrong"? The only thing you can do "wrong" as a mother is to be abusive in language and deed.

That aside, in the whole history of motherhood, there has yet to be a mother who hasn't unintentionally screwed up on something; this includes your own mother, and look how well you turned out!

Need more reassurance? Learn as much about parenting as you can. Start with the chapter, "Reality Bites," in this book.

3. Need for privacy

The second top reason for delaying motherhood, a loss of privacy, is a real concern when you have kids (if only I had a quarter for every mother of little ones who told me, "Oh, how I wish I could have the bathroom to myself just once").

Admittedly, finding private time is much more of a challenge while the kids are still toddling around the house or small enough to want to include you in every new thought and adventure when they are home from school. Mothers since time immemorial have gotten through this period of mothering. You will, too, with a little help from your friends. Trade off an afternoon with another mother from playgroup or hire a teenager to play with your child while you catch up on some phone calls.

Also, your child will need down time as well. With all the stimuli surrounding him or her, your child needs privacy as much—and maybe more—than you do.

And count your blessings: Two women in their eighties told me that as mothers of young children they rarely were able to leave the house—no car, limited public transportation, no lightweight, portable strollers that can be opened with one hand, no disposable diapers and wipes to make leaving the house easier—and most unbelievable of all—no neighborhood malls to wander.

Baby, Oh Midlife Baby: Thirty-Two Questions to Help You Decide, Compiled from Those Who Have Been There

Forethought is everything. The following questions were devised from a variety of resources, including lots of later-in-life moms. While some questions may make you feel defeated before you start, they are intended to help you think through the realities rather than give up. Becoming a mother at this point in your life is enough reward for some possible trade-offs.

1. **How strong is your longing to mother?** Do you feel you will miss out on a full life if you don't become a mother at this point in your life? Does your desire increase with the passage of time?

2. **What about your partner, if there is one?** How does he feel about having children at this stage of his life? Is his desire as strong as yours?

3. **Are you in a stable relationship?** Do you and your husband and/or partner have lots of separate interests or do you enjoy doing things together as a family? Do you think a child will fix a soured marriage/relationship? How well do you handle conflict? Do you have similar lifestyle desires?

4. **Do you like being with children in their world?** This is a different consideration than "do you like children?" When you have children of your own, you will be spending lots of time—especially at the beginning—with your child. Do you like making sand castles, camping, crawling on your knees to see where the ant is going, getting frosting in your hair as well as on your kitchen walls? Or are you strictly an art gallery and fine-dining kind of gal?

5. **Are you open to a different path to mothering than you've envisioned as "perfect"?** If you aren't able to get pregnant (75 percent of women over thirty-five have some infertility problems), how do you feel about:*

   A) Using another woman's egg?
   B) Using a sperm donor?
   C) Surrogacy?
   D) Adoption?
   E) Foster mothering?

6. **Are you willing to possibly go through very close medical scrutiny by your ob/gyn?** Would you be willing to follow what might be limiting instructions in order to bring a baby to full term?

7. **What if an amniocentesis showed your fetus had Down's syndrome?** What would you want to do? How does your partner feel about this possibility?

8. **What about twins, triplets or . . . ?** Even without fertility drugs, the chances for multiple births increase as you age. What will life be like with more than one crying infant at a time or more than one teenage daughter going through her first romance?

9. **Are you part of the sandwich generation?** Extra physical and mental energy is needed to care for an elderly parent and child at the same time. There

---

Each of these options is considered in detail later in this book.

might also be an increase in your monthly outgo to help pay expenses.

10. **What preexisting obligations do you have?** Don't think of this consideration only in terms of money. For instance, have you committed to a project that is going to keep you away from home?

11. **What kind of parent(s) would you make?** What strengths and weaknesses would you bring to the job? What about your partner's qualities? Do the two of you see eye-to-eye on how a child should be raised? One mother says a good test question to ask each other is, "How would you feel if our son wanted to pierce his nose or our daughter wanted to drop out of school?"

12. **What is your messiness tolerance level?** How important is a neat, orderly home? Do you take pride in having a place for everything and everything in its place? How do you feel about other people touching your personal things?

13. **What about noise?** Do you look forward to coming home to the silence of your home? Can you envision coming home instead to the blare of a toy fire truck and a two-year-old in the throes of a temper tantrum?

14. **How flexible are you?** Are you able to change course in midstream and go with the flow of the moment, or do

friends tell you that you are set in your ways? Children of all ages have short attention spans that you'll need to reconcile with your tolerance for flexibility.

15. **Are you creative?** Mothering is a matter of creating all the time: creating things for your bored children to do, creating ways to teach your child the ABCs, creating ways to guide them through valuable life lessons.

16. **How is your general health?** When was the last time you got a checkup? Any potential concerns that need to be attended to?

17. **Do you tire easily?** This is one of the biggest concerns of midlife mothers. The real question is: Do you have enough energy to escort a small child up and down the slide fourteen times in a row?

18. **What are your health and fitness habits?** Do you work out regularly, or hike or walk briskly on a regular basis? Is strength training included in your routine?

19. **How satisfied are you with your life as it is now?** If you are very satisfied now, how will adding a child to your life add to that satisfaction?

20. **Will you be isolated in your community?** If you live in a smaller community where most of the mothers are probably younger, are you self-contained enough

to be the only older mother in your playgroup? See more about this in the "Reality Bites" chapter.

21. **How will a child affect your current friendships?** Many women report a change in the status of their old friendships with women who are either childless like they were, or who are already grandparents.

22. **How important are other people's opinions?** How will you handle other people's proclamations about your decision? Friends? Family? Strangers?

23. **How are you at making long-term commitments?** You cannot divorce or leave a child—or trade your child in or get a refund. Motherhood lasts a lifetime.

24. **Can you put your family's needs and goals ahead of yours?** Are you able to put your immediate gratification on the shelf because your child's needs should come first? Are you willing to forgo some of the interests you love in order to give your child time with his or her interests?

25. **Can you handle the extra day-to-day expenses?** Toys, Mommy 'n' Me classes, music lessons, swim lessons, as well as medical expenses, clothes and day care all cost money.

26. **How is your income serving you in your present circumstances?** Is there room for more than the necessities once a child comes along, or will you be struggling to tighten your belt? While finances alone

should not be a deterrent to motherhood, it is a factor that needs to be figured into the mix.

27. **What career decisions do you need to rework to accommodate a new life?** Will you stay home full-time, work outside of the house or create a new option? Read the chapter entitled, "Do You Work?" to consider your choices.

28. **If one of you stays at home to parent full time, can you make do with one source of income?** "Becoming a mother later on requires planning and forethought," warns one fifty-four-year-old mother of two teenaged boys.

29. **Are you financially prepared to handle college tuition for your child and retirement for you at the same time?** The good news is that it is not too late to talk to a financial planner if you haven't started a savings program yet. It's also important to not panic about college for your child just now. First you have to get through kindergarten.

30. **Is your present home large enough to accommodate a new family member?** Will you have to move? How will that affect the rest of the family?

31. **Are you good at setting up a support system for yourself?** New moms of any age may need help getting their feet wet (at least in the beginning). Start now to think about how to arrange family and friend support.

32. **Will you enjoy having someone totally dependent on you for a few years?** At the beginning, your infant relies on you for every bodily function as well as his or her well-being, warmth, security and happiness. As your child grows, he or she will need your hands-on input less and less; but motherhood remains a lifelong proposition. Which is also the good news.

The Decision to Restart Motherhood: Go Forth and Multiply—or Maybe Not

In 1998, of the women who were "through with the childbearing years" (according to the National Center for Health Statistics), 17.5 percent had only one child. That shows a remarkable 10 percent increase in single-child families over the decade before. The research concluded that children born to older mothers (especially women over forty) are likely to be only children.

It makes sense. Women who marry for the first time later in life start families later in life and have less of a chance or desire to parent more than one child.

Divorce has also contributed to single-child families. In the past few decades, the incidence of divorce is the highest it's ever been; this increases the likelihood that a couple might separate before they have an opportunity to expand the family they already have. In the early 1900s, divorce was a rarity, as were small families: Not only did it take every hand to keep the family farm running, birth control was not plentifully available.

Single Children Do Not "Need" Siblings . . .

Moreover, the perception of an only child being "lonely" or "spoiled" has proven unfounded. A University of Texas study concurs: Only children are not maladjusted. On the contrary, they are higher achievers in school and often have better self-images than their sibling-laden peers. They are frequently included in their parents' grown-up conversations and therefore get a jump-start on adult vocabulary. Because they don't have built-in playmates, only children are more likely to rely on their own imagination. They are secure, stable, socially sensitive and no more likely to be shy than children who have siblings. Finally, in the last part of the twentieth century, researchers stopped hearing terms such as "selfish" in discussions about only children.

"We can do so much more for him than if he had a brother or sister. And I don't mean just monetarily, but with our time, attention and interest," reasons one forty-six-year-old mother of a seven-year-old.

"Now there are two soccer practices—not to mention two games—each week. I have to volunteer two times a week in school, drive them to two piano lessons. It all falls on me to transport them everywhere—or make sure arrangements are made to get them around—and then I have to follow through to make sure those arrangements are carried out, carried out safely and on time. Oh, did I mention that in addition, even though I work from home, I work full time?" another mother, with two active daughters, nine and eleven, bemoaned. "I love my daughters, but I am sometimes envious of my friends with one child."

But on the Other Hand, Single Children *Do* Need Siblings

What about the empty space you, your partner or other children are feeling that hasn't been filled by a new puppy or a world cruise? This particular longing can only be filled by another child.

"I am so much more tired with two. There is rarely any time for my partner and myself alone. We always have something that needs to be done. My energy is rapidly vanishing—and sometimes my patience. But when you ask me if I would have wanted another child if I knew what was involved? You bet!" a happy new-again midlife mother reports.

While it makes sense that women who marry later in life may not have had a chance before their marriage to start a family, it's also true that midlife couples who have stayed together through the raising of the first child(ren) may want to restart a family; the older children have less time for their parents, but the parents miss that hands-on parenting of a young child. This may be more true of women than men. Just because a woman's birth certificate is getting a little dog-eared doesn't mean she's lost the desire to be a mommy.

Single children could be at risk for having a harder time adjusting to the socialization that is a primary part of school or day care. A child with no siblings is used to being the center of the universe. One preschool director who's an older mom herself said she can always tell which children come from homes with no siblings at the beginning of the school term: It's the difference between a child who has to share at home and one who doesn't.

This risk is one reason to join a playgroup, no matter how many siblings your child has. (See the chapter entitled "Reality Bites" for more information on playgroups).

Are You Raising the Future Sandwich Generation?

As children of older parents, our sons and daughters might be trapped in their sandwich generation years at a much younger age than many of their peers. Do we want our only child to carry the burden of caring for us by themselves? "I used to think this was a selfish way to see having another child, a sort of nonsensical reason to become a mother again. But the truth is that while it *was* a factor in deciding to have another baby, we love our second son and can't imagine what life would be like without him. He's not just a sibling for our other son," a fifty-one-year-old mother of a four-year-old and eighteen-month-old says.

Some of the Reasons Mothers Want to Start Motherhood All Over Again

- Starting over with a new relationship
- Looking for a new start in the same long-time relationship
- Tired of their work career
- Newly single
- New view of life
- No longer *have* to work full time
- "Everyone else" has two kids but her
- A feeling it's her "last chance"
- An opportunity to do some parenting things differently: "It's such a blessing to be able to correct mistakes I made with the first child."

Considering Another Child in Midlife

A new child comes with a new set of circumstances no matter if your other child(ren) are grown and out of the house or still tottering around in diapers. This is especially true for women who are over thirty-five and forty *for all the same considerations this book has been looking at.*

In addition to the thirty-two point questionnaire on page forty-one, here are some points to consider when thinking of increasing your family size again:

1. **What are the ages of the other children living at home?** Are they old enough to help out with a new addition to the family? How much do they need you?

2. **How do you envision your family life will change with another child?** Will you have to make sacrifices if you have another child? This can include parenting as well as lifestyle.

3. **Would it be a strain on your family if you gave birth to more than one child?** Remember, there is a higher incidence of multiple births in older women whether or not they have gone through fertility treatments.

4. **Will you be a new mother and grandmother at the same time?** How can you balance both roles so everyone (including you) wins?

5. **Why do you want another child?** Are you looking for a playmate for your only child? If so, join a playgroup.

"I Love My Child So Much, I Can't Imagine Loving Another One."

It's a little talked-about sentiment, yet many women feel concerned they won't love a new child as much as they love the one(s) they already have. This concern appears to be widespread and normal; for the vast majority of new-again mothers, it becomes a nonissue once their new child is home.

Here's a response that is fairly reflective of mothers who started over in midlife. It comes from a fifty-year-old mother of a two-year-old and a seven-year-old: "I truly didn't feel as if I had room to love again the way I loved my first son. I'll admit it took a little while longer to fall in love with my second child, but I can't ever imagine not having him now. He makes such a difference in our lives and we *all* love him so much."

What's Right for You?

In the end, a Loyola University study found that family size is irrelevant when it comes to how happy the parents are; the determining factor is what is right for each individual family.

A Personal Note

At times, I spy women my own age watching Skyler and myself; they look as if they question the veracity of my sanity. I admit it: Sometimes I, too, question my own sanity in becoming a mother after all those perfectly agreeable years childless.

Those moments are so very, very few. And they diminish totally in the face of the swelled-up fulfillment I feel in the center of my being since his arrival in my life.

And a Warning

Now that you've made the decision to forge ahead, be forewarned. At times you will feel like you are being blown about like a sail on a boat as you flap helplessly between disappointments and fulfilled expectations— especially if you are going through infertility or adoption. Hang onto the mast, for although your quest to become an older mother can be a wild ride, once you land, it will feel like you have come home at last.

One Last Point

Your decision to start or restart a family is personal, but if it's a go, it needs to be acted on, especially if your decision includes trying to get pregnant. The single loudest regret one hears from midlife mothers is that they didn't act sooner.

CHAPTER 5

What Kids of Later-in-Life Mothers Have to Say About Having Later-in-Life Mothers

A study conducted by the University of Southern California over a period of a quarter of a century proffered a remarkable conclusion: In many important ways, older parents are better parents.

Gerontology and Sociology Professor Vern L. Bengtson says, "These kids are desired and planned for. Their nursery and pre-kindergarten days have been more carefully attended than perhaps any other children in history."

Despite these encouraging findings, women who are considering becoming a mother beyond the so-called traditional years some-times feel that they will embarrass their child by being the oldest member of the PTA; they also some-times feel it is selfish to have children at an older age since they might not have as much energy as younger parents, or that they might die while their children are still young.

But according to research, there are many strong advan-tages (see the Pros and Cons chapter). One big plus is that they had time to work through their own "issues" to be able to center their lives unselfishly and without resentment on their children.

So, just how do kids of older mothers fare in a time when the ages of mothers are all over the map—as well as the park and the PTA?

Since adults often rush in to speak for children, here, in the kids' own words, are what children say it's like to have an older mommy:

"My mother is the coolest one of all my friends' mothers.
All my friends are jealous."

CATHY, AGE 8

"Sometimes I worry that my mother will die
before the other mothers. But my mother told me that
people can die at any age and that she couldn't guarantee
anything, but that she was very healthy and planned
to stay that way because of me."

JASON, AGE 9

"If I got to do everything I wanted to do,
I guess that wouldn't be good either. At least my
parents always take time to tell me why,
not like some of my friends' parents."

CYNTHIA, AGE 12

"I disagree with how my fifty-two-year-old
mother is raising her two children (seven and three).
She went back to work soon after they were born.
Why have them so late in life if you are going to
put them in day care all day? I also worry that she
won't be there to be a grandmother to my kids,
let alone a mother to her own."

ELISA, 25, MOTHER OF THREE

"My parents were the ones who always
had time and interest in me way more than my
friends' parents did. Perhaps because they
already had established careers."

ALAIN, AGE 17

"I was miserable and embarrassed growing up
with older parents. They never let me do the things
other kids could do. I couldn't even go to
dances with lots of other kids."

DEBRA, AGE 15

"My parents aren't workaholics.
They have more time to play with me,
and we go lots of places together."

ROBERT, AGE 9

"I think it's great! My forty-seven-year-old
mother has a two-year-old son, and so do I. She stays
home with both of them, and they are like brothers.
No one makes a big deal out of it.
She got pregnant by surprise, and it gave her
a whole new lease on life. She's also a lot more
patient and doesn't worry as much about things like
when she raised us. She's having a blast."

MARK, 27

"Both my parents were older than
everyone else's in my class. When I was really little
I didn't know. When I started to realize that my mother
looked older, she told me that she waited to have a
really special baby, which turned out to be me.
Still, I was sometimes embarrassed.
Now, of course, I realize that all kids are
embarrassed by their parents about
something or other."

LUCY, 17

*"My friends' moms are always busy working,
so they don't have time to come to their basketball games.
Maybe they are the ones who shouldn't have kids!
My mom always tells me that I am her priority."*

ANGEL, 11

*"I don't see that it makes any difference.
What counts is if your parents love you or not."*

MARJORIE ANNE, 9

*"They always knew what I was doing.
Their entire attention was focused on me, and
I couldn't get away with things like some of my friends could.
Now that I'm a parent myself, I can see why they did it
that way; but as a teenager, I hated them for it.
Why couldn't they be too busy to ignore me
like my friends' parents?"*

JUDY, 26

*"My sisters were a lot older and out of the house
when I came along. It was great.
I never had to share my parents with them."*

CECI, 21

*"We went on a lot of trips, more so than my friends did.
My parents wanted us to learn about different cultures
firsthand, but they traveled for themselves as well.
They didn't wait until we were 'old enough'
by everyone else's standards."*

GAIL, 28

*"I wouldn't like to have an older mother.
I'd rather have you."*

SKYLER, 5

CHAPTER 6

More Mommyhood: Single, Step- and Lesbian Mothering

W omen who delay raising children have sometimes spent their time building complex and not-so-traditional lives prior to coming to motherhood.

For single, lesbian and stepmothers, here are some special considerations for this new phase of their lives.

Single Mothering

When the unmarried TV character Murphy Brown became pregnant past the age of forty, she stirred up a lot of controversy hurled at women raising children on their own. Despite those charges (or maybe because of them), the numbers of women heading households increased each year to where there are almost 16 million kids in the United States now living in single-parent households, mainly with mothers.

Many of these women got tired of waiting for Mr. Right to come along before they could parent; others who were once married now live separately from their child's father.

Whether by choice or circumstance, if your child grows up in a single-parent home, she will not be alone: 61 percent of single women surveyed in 2000 by *Time* magazine said that if circumstances warranted, they would definitely raise a child on their own.

"I would try to talk myself out of things in the past," says one single mom, thirty-eight, with a two-year-old girl. "Now I realize I am capable, and I have put together resources and support. And I have so much to give."

Being a single parent can be overwhelming. First of all, there's the economic factor: Holding up the financial end by yourself means planning. Can your present state of income and finances carry that burden to your satisfaction? Many single moms without these resources find that life can be challenging. Plan now to avoid these problems. Also, taking care of a child completely by yourself, through thick and thin, sickness and health—not to mention soccer practice—is an enormous job. "I'm resourceful," says one mom. "But in some regards, it's also easier. I see married friends struggling with parenting perspectives that differ from their partners'. I don't have that issue."

Craving a child and finally getting one is a special trea-sure for single older mothers. "I can't worry about what other people think. I knew I'd make a very good mother, and it happens that I am also single," a forty-five-year-old single mom determines.

"Now when I come home from work, I have someone to come home to, someone who is excited to see me aside from the dog," says another very happy over-forty mother of a toddler son.

Finding Support

If you are a single mother, realize that you are an inde-pendent woman capable of doing many things on your own; however, gathering support when needed is never a bad idea. In the beginning, when so many things need to be tended to at once, set yourself up with at least one other parent you can rely on for trade-off relief when you need it. You've got to take breaks for your own sanity. Use the time to take a bath, go for a walk, have a cup of java in total, total peace. Try to choose someone who might look for-ward to being a long-term hands-on "auntie or uncle" and/or someone whose parenting style you respect.

If there is no one like this in your immediate circle, con-sider hiring a baby-sitter or nanny. "You can't blame others for not helping," one realistic single mom determines.

Finding Male "Role Models" for Your Child

Being around a male personality your child can emulate is an important part of every child's development. Men and women are different; ergo they bring different qualities to the table. The need for male figures in your child's life shows up in unforeseen big and small ways: "Now that he's potty training, I admit I wish my son had a guy around to show him where to aim. So, I ask guy friends who are understanding," a single mom with a three-year-old reports.

Ask male friends and relatives to chip in with their time; trade-off the concept with a single dad in need of a woman's influence at home. In lieu of these choices, register your child with Big Brothers/Big Sisters, find a male teacher or coach, or ask someone at your job or place of spiritual worship to commit to spending time with your child.

But do not think the fact that your child has no everyday father in the picture will hinder his or her development into a fully functioning adult: "As for men in her life," a thirty-seven-year-old single mom of a one-year-old daughter ponders, "I came to wonder, are we after role models of how to be a man or how to be a good human being, period?"

Letting Go of Guilt

There are only so many hours in a day and only so many things you can accomplish in those hours. Wasting time feeling bad that you haven't "done it all" for your child is just that—wasting time. That includes feeling guilty over your child not having a dad living at home.

If you start to beat yourself up, heed the advice of one single-by-choice mother, forty-two, with a four-year-old child: "I'm a better mom on my own than I would be if I was in a lousy relationship."

Advice from Single Moms Over Thirty-Five and Forty

- "Hire someone to do housework so you have more time with your child. If you can't afford it, lower your housekeeping standards."

- "Be careful not to overstep the boundary between parent and buddy, or worse yet, make your child into a substitute partner as I did. When it's just the two of you palling around together, it's hard to stop and say to yourself, 'Wait a minute. I'm the parent here.' On the other hand, you have a wonderful opportunity to develop a very strong bond between just the two of you, without other family members around. It's a tradeoff and an opportunity married mothers don't get."

- "In addition to making sure you spend a focused block of time with your child each day, give yourself some focused time in a solo retreat."

- "Find other single parents to commiserate with and befriend you."

Lesbian Mothering

Another type of mothering that requires working at balancing the male–female role modeling is lesbian mothering. Well-known older lesbian moms include comedian-actress Sandra Bernhard, who, at forty-three became a mom. Perhaps the most well-publicized celebrity lesbian mother is singer Melissa Etheridge, who, in late 1999, revealed that friend and rock singer, David Crosby, contributed sperm—twice—so her partner could become pregnant.

Melissa was in her mid- and then again in her later thirties when she became a mother.

"I tell our daughter there are lots of different kinds of families," Etheridge said in an interview. "Some families have a mommy and daddy, some have just a mommy, some have two mommies. . . . I believe in giving kids the truth."

Commonly in lesbian relationships, the pair chooses one of the women to get pregnant via donor sperm or to adopt; later on, the other parent will adopt the child where that can be legally accomplished. In cases when the other mother cannot legally adopt the child, it is advised to consult a lawyer to make certain that the nonlegal mother has rights to her child if something happens to the legal mother. This is also a wise decision if the mothers' families are adverse to the arrangement and might try to block contact by the non-legal mother in the event of an accident or death of the legal mother.

The Role of Men in Your Child's Life

So many stereotypes exist about lesbians. One of the most unfounded is that if a woman is a lesbian she must hate men. "This is simply illogical. Just because I love a woman romantically, doesn't mean I can't love men in nonromantic ways," one fifty-two-year-old lesbian mother declares.

"I'm glad I have a son. Fifty percent of the world are men," another mother in a lesbian relationship says. Her partner concurs: "I don't have to raise him in a female-only world just because there are no men living in my house." As for getting more male perspective into your child's life, read the advice for single moms in this chapter.

More Misconceptions About Lesbian Mothering

- "Just as there is a misconception that lesbians hate men, there is a misconception about lesbians and daughters: Since we aren't 'real' women, we won't know how to raise 'real' girls. That's as nonsensical as the belief that lesbians can only raise gay boys and lesbian girls. My parents weren't homosexual, so how is that explained?" This mother also said that when her daughter was a mere five months old, people would ask if the child was gay.

- "My mother was very upset that I got pregnant with an unknown sperm donor; she would lie and tell other family members made-up stories about how I got pregnant—including that I was raped. But since our daughter was born, she's done a complete turn-around. They are even polite to my partner of twenty years."

- One forty-one-year-old reported that she and her partner waited past the first trimester to tell their families, bracing themselves for a negative reaction. "We were expecting lots of family anger; instead, both of our mothers keep pushing us to do it again!"

How Lesbian Moms See Their Decision to Have Children Later in Life:

- "At first I was concerned about what people would think of me. Then I realized I wasn't some teenager who had gotten pregnant by accident."

- "This was something I had given a lot of thought to. My partner of almost fifteen years and I had researched the idea," says one forty-eight-year-old mother of a two-year-old boy.

- Her partner adds: "I'm a very good mother, and it happens that coincidentally I am a lesbian. I can't help what other people think."

- "I got pregnant because I wanted to parent, just like anybody else—not to raise a clone of ourselves," another lesbian mom chimes in.

- "My biggest fear is how my child's friends will react to him having two mommies—lesbians. I think it's key to choose an open-minded school and area to live in," a forty-two-year-old teacher and lesbian mother of a five-year-old son advises.

- "We are in a better situation than many traditional parents we know. One of us works, the other stays home to attend to our boys' needs," says a fifty-year-old mother of two adopted sons, five and one. "Most other lesbian couples we know have the same arrangement. There are lots of stay-at-home moms *by choice* who also happen to be lesbians."

Stepmothering

According to the Stepfamily Association of America, a stepfamily is formed when a parent marries a person who is not his or her child's other parent. Since the Census Bureau only counts children where they actually live full time (and generally that means with the original mom), there are virtually no statistics to show how many stepmoms are out there. With that in mind, it is known that stepfamilies are the fastest-growing type of family (one-quarter of kids under eighteen are a stepchild to someone). In large part, stepfamilies are formed as the result of divorce and remarriage, traditionally the territory of women over thirty-five and beyond forty.

What Is a Typical Stepfamily?

The typical form a stepfamily takes is . . . well, there is no typical form for a stepfamily. They can all live under the same roof year-round, shuttle from home to home (mainly the children do the shuttling), be children only of one or the other parent, or each partner can bring their children from past relationships into the mix. In addition, new children are many times borne out of the new marriage.

Working with, Not Against, Your New Mate

Many women who waited for motherhood eye a man who already has kids as a great catch: They get the man and the cute little *grateful* cherubs all in one. Instant family. The reality is that just because you are married to their dad, doesn't mean the kids will accept you as their mom, even if their own mom is no longer in the picture.

The relationship between your husband, your husband's ex-wife and their children has been around a lot longer than your relationship with any of them. Stepmothers in the know advise really taking time to get to know the kids' dad before jumping into marriage. Will he support you in front of his kids as well as behind your back? By showing his respect for you, the kids will learn to respect you as well. If you are always in disagreement about the kids, chances arc you will be the one who will be the wicked (step)parent, not him—and probably not their mother.

Working with, Not Against, the Ex

Handling the logistics of schooling, traveling between homes, family finances, vacation holidays and stepsibling rivalry can be a full-time job. What makes it especially hard is that a stepparent is generally at the mercy of agreements worked out between her new spouse and his old spouse; the stepmother usually has no legal relationship to the children. She is not the legal mom, adoptive mom or a foster mom—she is "only" the stepmom.

On a practical level, this legal state of mothering limbo must be addressed directly. What if your stepchild breaks his leg in a basketball game while he is in your care? The emergency room nurse may need information you can't provide—assuming you were even allowed to have a say in how the child should be cared for.

By asking your husband and his ex-wife to grant you a limited power of attorney for emergency medical care, you can head this kind of situation off. It will allow you to do your best under the worst kinds of conditions without worrying about stepping over your boundaries. Hopefully, your husband's ex-wife will realize that it is to her children's advantage to accept you as a fact of everyone's life.

If she is at all evolved (and she must be since she once fell in love with the same man you did), she can see the trade-off in respecting your new role: You will similarly respect her in her physical absence.

Disciplining in Stepfamilies: Who and How

Stepfamilies often experience discipline as more of a challenge than other families. A good rule of thumb to follow, at least at first, is that when it comes to disciplining his kids, *he* should be the ultimate decision-maker about what they can and cannot do, say, wear, etc. But these kids are also living in your home. *Your* marriage and your mothering also needs respect.

The disciplining scenario can start something like this: Your husband dispenses the actual discipline to the children, but with your agreement of what that will look like (e.g., bedtime by 9:00 P.M. on school nights). Then, as time goes on and trust has been built between you and your stepchildren, you can do some direct disciplining. In this way, the children will see you as someone they must also respect because their father does. If you try to discipline them from the get-go, more than likely the kids will ignore you—or worse. Ease into your new responsibilities: Attend after school activities with your stepchildren or drive them to and from friends' houses so you have a little time to talk together.

Always discuss discipline with your new husband when the kids aren't around; this is something smart to do whether or not you have stepchildren.

Is It Easier if Your Stepchildren Are Boys or Girls?

Both genders can present problems to the newly formed stepfamily. Girls, especially older ones, can be very close to their mothers and resentful of any mothering you might want to give—from picking out Halloween costumes to helping with homework. They might also see themselves as "Daddy's little girl" and resent your intrusion in that relationship.

Boys may also resent your intrusion in the special relationship that has been built between father and son. Older sons who are growing critical of their dads during their attempts to grow into separate young men may be suspicious: What would you want with *their* Dad?

Older Stepmothers Speak: The Realities

- "My husband's ex-wife actually told her kids not to talk to me—even when they were in my home. I didn't know this until, on our first visit, my husband's eight-year-old son and I were laughing together and he put his hand over his mouth. 'I forgot,' he said. 'I'm not supposed to talk to you.' He was afraid he was going to get into trouble."

- "Everyone—outside of myself and my husband anyway—acts as if our stepfamily is not a real family . . . that the only family that counts is the one with my husband's ex-wife. But, the kids live here for long periods of time. They are not just guests. So, it is a family."

- "Fall in love if you can't help yourself, but don't think marrying someone with kids from another marriage is a piece of cake. Your expectations of an automatic close-knit family life are likely to slap you in your face. It takes time and work, but it definitely can be worth it."

- "I made an assumption that we'd all get along and mix together easily in one big happy family sort of way. But this wasn't the movies. It took a long while to make it all work. We had four different personalities, four different needs, wants and thoughts about how we should use our diminishing funds, and four different ways we handle our feelings, all under one roof."

- "The kids and I didn't grow up together, so we had to hit the ground running. The worst part of it was as soon as we started to get into a rhythm, they were packing to go home to their mother."
- "I can feel left out when my husband and his children talk about vacations or other things that happened when I wasn't around."

Some Practical Tips and Some Things to Keep in Mind

- A stepfamily is formed as the result of some kind of loss: a divorce or death of a parent. The children must be allowed their grieving period, which can include anger directed at you. They are feeling a loss of stability as well as the loss of their dream of what it meant to have their own mother and father under one roof.
- Just because your husband was ready to move on doesn't mean that his children were ready. Give it time.
- Care for yourself in this mix. Take mini-breaks away for a few hours or a day if it gets too hard.
- Try to arrange alone time with each child in order to do things that you two can enjoy together; these can become the basis of a special relationship between you.
- Whether or not your husband's ex-wife is still living, tell your stepchildren that it is not your intention to replace her.

- Don't get hung up on what your stepchildren call you ("Mom," "Sara"), as long as it's respectful.

No Doubt . . .

Families that don't fall into the traditional categories—single, lesbian and stepmothering amongst them—can be an eye-opening challenge, in addition to the other later-in-life mothering challenges that exist. However, being a lesbian or single mother or stepmother (nontraditional ways to mother) in combination with being older (another nontraditional way to mother) will not combine to create a third special circumstance that needs to be contended with.

The majority of these less-traditional families are working it out to the benefit of all members. Armed with a little support and some knowledge of what to expect, there is no doubt yours will also work—and more than that, be a very enriching circumstance in your life.

CHAPTER 7

Reality Bites (And Kicks and Screams and Says "No, Mommy! No!"): What Life Is *Really* Like for the Midlife Mommy

T oo often women who delay growing a family are so wrapped up in the process of getting a child that they don't take time to think about what their daily lives will be like once their child arrives. Until I held Skyler in my arms the first time and tasted the tears I was surprised sprung up so spontaneously, I had no clue nor any interest in "parenting." I thought it was just another tired buzzword. I believed that because I loved him so heart-achingly much, it'd all work out: you know, that he'd just come along with us in whatever we were doing, like wine tasting or dining at restaurants that don't hand you your dinner in a bag as you drive by. That sort of thing.

Picture this much naiveté coming out of the mouth of your teenage daughter in regard to a subject like her boyfriend. You wouldn't think twice about locking her in her room until she was, oh, say forty, when she would have developed enough common sense since, after all, she would be a mid-age adult. Or so one would presume.

The biggest eye-opener for first-time middle-year mothers is that children come with their own agendas, agendas that have a way of taking over everyone else's, especially yours. Now, I can hear you saying: "But, I've always planned my life down to the last detail (aside from forgetting to have children). There's no reason why my life can't be just as organized after I become a mother, too."

Ha.

The bare truth is no one can tell you what it is like to be a mother until you are one. No matter how many little nieces and nephews or friends' kids call you "auntie," having your own child is different (it's much better). From the moment your child comes home, your life will be forever changed (it's much more magical). From that moment on, no matter how carefully you plot out a schedule (we'll leave the house by 8:15 A.M.), your child has his or her own plans (okay, 9:30 A.M.; he or she needed a last-minute diaper change).

If I had to bet on whose agenda wins, my money is on your child's. As one very astute later-in-life mother points out, "Women who wait to have children learn quickly that even the most cautious planning goes into the wastebasket once kids come along."

Adding a baby to the family means decorating will take on a whole new significance. You will learn to accessorize around a playpen with that infamous pink doll motif or choo-choo train.

Clothes shopping will be limited to a wash-and-wear wardrobe that goes with sticky fingers (this applies to yours as well as your child's). Laundry? Well, just as I never knew it was possible to love so deeply, so unconditionally, I never knew it was possible that one small child could create so much laundry or that I would have to tote so many extra bags filled with—stuff!?—on a simple trip to the bank.

You will amaze yourself at the things you suddenly think are cute; things your former nonparent self would consider unthinkable—nay, abominable. Like allowing your child to record the outgoing message on your answering machine, or even more unimaginable, answer your ringing phone directly, breathing-on but not quite talking-to whatever poor soul is dangling on the other end of the line. You will not think this obnoxious: You will think your child is a genius for learning to use the phone.

And at a time when you are finally able to afford the "adult" furnishings of your dreams, along comes your little one to paint her version of a Kadinsky (with chocolate-covered hands) all over your white silk duvet. "How clever!" you'll think. "Look at the variation in those lines."

Your life will move from fairly orderly to unimaginably extraordinary. Watching your own child grow, having an enormous influence over the way in which a whole human being develops intellectually, spiritually, physically, emotionally, socially, creatively—and then the icing on the cake, hearing your very own child say "I love you" totally unprompted.

Welcome to later-in-life motherhood. Can anything compare?

The Reality Comes Home: Women and Men Experience Parenthood Differently

Nature cleverly put us into middle life at a time when we are changing attitudes and priorities in many areas. Midlife is an epiphany; roles shift and we have an opportunity to intensely explore the meaning of our lives. We examine what we want to get rid of, as well as what we'd like to add to our lives. It's not surprising that children are a major part of this rethinking, especially if a woman has not mothered yet, it's been a long time since she had small ones or she got started late and wants siblings for her other child. Perhaps a child is the perfect way to connect this phase of her life with the next.

Women Who Delay Motherhood Often "Glamorize" Family Life

Have you given thought yet to how motherhood will look on you? What will be different about your life? Like many wanna-be later mothers, I had a picture in my mind of what motherhood would be like for me. I wandered the park on Sunday afternoons; where I lived at the time there were many "graying" mommies toting young babies. I hungered after the beautifully dressed cherubs sleeping softly in their strollers, soaking up the sun on their velvety cheeks. When I glanced at the mothers, their faces beamed with earned pride.

I couldn't wait. I even had the wardrobe picked out!

What I had failed to consider was how much work goes into getting a squirmy, fussy baby into a clean, adorable outfit that he hadn't outgrown overnight. That accomplished, the challenge becomes finding time to get showered and dressed myself with one hand while carrying a wailing baby with the other (only a new mother can appreciate what a luxury it is to be able to pull on her jeans using two hands).

Women who have waited to begin a family often envision parenting as warm hugs from small, clean children; they fail to extrapolate beyond that. They romanticize what their daily life will be once they become mothers. They push their long-held dream onto the grass where it is always "greener."

You've Come a Long Way Baby— Just Not Far Enough

Just as the division of labor in most relationships continues to fall mainly on the female, things are likewise unbalanced when it comes to parenting. While men now perform more of the so-called traditional activities, it remains the principal domain of the mother to be the activity director, teacher, transportation captain, nutritionist, therapist, activity participant and general life liaison. This, in addition to whatever else she was doing B.B. (Before Baby), including household chores.

Luckily, dreams definitely come true. More times than you can ever, ever imagine, you will be the recipient of your dreams: warm hugs and feathery soft kisses from a clean, adorably dressed happy child. It's just more than likely that you'll be the one doing the cleaning and the dressing.

Men Picture the First Ball Game Together

Okay, okay. This trivializes men and their parenting role, but it does underscore the difference in the nature of men and women and what each sees as important in the role of a parent.

Many men like to engage in rough-and-tumble play with their kids that frequently makes women cringe. It's a complaint heard over and over: "I'm trying to quiet our son down before sleep with classical music or a nice story. My husband thinks winding him down includes playing bed-time touch football." In his research on families, Dr. Scott Coltrane discovered that while this pattern sets many a mother's teeth on edge, it also serves a purpose:

"What this rough-and-tumble play does is teach a child to set limits on himself. This in turn makes children 'other focused' and makes them into more competent friends later in life," Dr. Coltrane told me. In addition, men use this technique as a way to show affection and bond with their children.

Men also differ in pre-planning what kind of parent they will be: basically, in greater numbers than women, well, they don't plan, they just "are." Women, on the other hand, are more prone to read everything they can find on parenting and plan what they should do. So, while you are obsessing over what your child will need to be nourished, comfortable and intellectually stimulated, your child's dad figures he'll have some little pal to shoot hoops with. This could explain why some men don't jump in with both feet until the child starts to walk and talk (not to suggest that they don't love them until then as much as you do; they just might not be as interested in the baby-phase as much as you are).

Admittedly, this oversimplifies the matter, but at some point, there is every chance your child's father will tell you that you worry about every detail of your child's life "too much."

The good news is that no matter how hair-pulling this scenario may seem to you, this yin-yang tug helps us turn out well-balanced children. (*Note:* If you are a mom with no dad in the house, see the chapter on "More Mommyhood" for ideas on how to get this type of balance in your home.)

Sigh. It Will Be Love at First Sight

Maybe. Maybe not. If you do not feel a tug on your heart strings the minute his adorable face is shown to you, do not panic. You might be like many mothers who don't experience instant love; give yourself some time. Maybe you are postpartum, which can happen to you whether you gave birth or adopted: The baby blues can come from feeling overwhelmed or facing everyday life again after the "high" you've just experienced knowing you were about to become a mother. (*Note:* If this a concern, seek professional help).

Before you know it, chances are you will be so in love you will find it hard to remove your gaze from your child's face long enough to brush your hair. And you will continue to fall in love over and over for a lifetime, just as you might with your husband.

Parenting Today Is Different than When Your Mother Mothered You

For one thing, nobody referred to it as "parenting." Our mothers relied more on instinct, less on step-by-step books, graphs, charts and workshops. Today, however, we live in information-saturated times. The mid-1990s, in particular, was a turning point. That's when we discovered how the brain develops from zero to age three and what the time-lines are for encouraging a propensity for language, math, music and more. Mothering is intensified these days as a result, and older mothers, especially, hit the ground running to ensure that their baby's neurons and synapses are firing to their maximum potential. You can't spend a day in the playground or at baby gym without hearing the phrase, "Their brains are like little sponges," followed by a discussion about how best to stimulate them.

As older mothers, we can feel anxious to make up for time lost; we desire to give our kids everything at once. We are more concerned with options for the right nutrition, playdates, toys, day care, clothes and appropriate discipline than our mothers ever thought existed. And why not? We have the resources, time and desire to put all our attention on our child. As a generation, we have had to compete in making a new world for ourselves. We want our kids to benefit, and benefit quickly. We may be calmer when the kids spill milk on the carpet, but we have a tendency to "push" our children, especially if he or she is an only child.

Playing is a child's job. Talk and read to your baby frequently. Walk with your baby in the stroller as you describe the falling leaves and changing seasons. Sing songs and play lovely music. Expose your child to lots of color. Rest assured that your child will lead you to his or her next stage of development when he or she is ready.

Just be prepared to follow along.

Is There Sex After Motherhood? (And Other Ways Your Life Will Change)

Life B.B. (Before Baby): Life B.B. are the days when the words "relationship," "career" and "spontaneous" were the centerpieces of your vocabulary. They are the days when free time exists to get together with your old friends (also probably childless or with grown children), take flute lessons *and* practice, go hiking or mountain biking, participate in after-work get-togethers, indulge in leisurely rambles through the mall, see a movie *and* have dinner out.

Life B.B. is a time when your gray matter is available to focus mainly on yourself.

Life A.C. (After Child): The other day I came across a card that I had given my husband on our first married

Valentine's Day: It reminisced about long Sunday break-
fasts, reading in bed together, casual strolls through the
park and rooms full of laughter. Now that we are parents,
the only thing true about that card is the rooms full of
laughter—and that's mainly true because our son is probably in the room and we are laughing at his antics.

"Children can be more of a disruption to the life of a
woman who delayed family life than to a younger one,"
says Dr. Coltrane. Older mothers and their partners have
been more ensconced in their old lifestyle longer than
younger mothers have. Even what we hunger for (like a
child) can be a challenge to which we must adjust. The
truth is, while there is that 1 percent who needs no sleep,
most older moms find they can't do it all and take care of
the baby, too. There are still only twenty-four hours a day,
seven days a week (and no time off for Thanksgiving). A
forty-two-year-old mother of three told me she never
remembers sighing before she had kids. "What I do
remember is occasionally laying down on the couch just
for the heck of it. Now I pass my couch and wink at it with
a knowing, 'Hey, remember me? I'll be with you again
someday, I hope.'"

Aside from filling your spare time with the physical
requirements of your new role, you'll find that your head is
generally filled with someone else's voice and needs as well.
Somehow, too, especially at the beginning of your motherhood, others will forget to ask how you are and go directly

to asking about your child. When they finally do get around to you, you will answer in terms of your child anyway as in, "Well, I'm feeling much better now that she no longer has a cough."

One often-overlooked way things will be different for you is in your present friendships. "What happened here?" one forty-three-year-old mother of two boys, six and two and a half, asked rhetorically. "I used to have such great girlfriends. Now I hardly see them anymore." Several things take place that can cause shifts in your old friendships: First of all, there is the time factor—there is much less of it. Second, it might surprise you to find out that your childless friends (especially) aren't excited to talk about your baby's poop. Third—and probably this is the biggest factor—you will lose interest in some of your old acquaintances as your new life opens to you. As a part of that natural course, you will also find new friends that you have more in common with for this stage of your life.

In relating to your true old friends, becoming a new mother will cut the wheat from the chaff because true friends never vanish; they just metamorphose into "aunties".

S-E-X? What's T-H-A-T?

Recent forays into the workings of romance found that sexual relations and satisfaction drops about 40 percent in the first year after baby comes home. This research is backed up by a survey compiled by *Parenting Magazine* showing couples are twice as likely to kiss their new baby as they are each other.

Our own totally unscientific polling discovered that there is a 99.99 percent chance (or more) that your personal private kissy-face relationship with your spouse will take an immediate (and willing) backseat to what has come to be known as the "child-centered" life.

There can be more than one reason for this phenomenon. One mother who waited says her relationship shifted because she felt her husband, used to it being just the two of them for many years, was jealous when her attentions focused more heavily on what the baby was doing rather than on her sulking husband. Another admits she "second guesses" the way her husband takes care of their long-waited-for child. He greets her criticism as a lack of confidence in him, rather than "maternal instincts in bloom."

Still another feels the loss of connection she and her spouse shared B.B. "The playfulness we once had with each other now goes to our kids," she says. Many older mothers typically felt like this forty-three-year-old mother of twin girls, age six: "We tried having date night like the magazines suggest, but we were either too tired to make love, or wound up talking about the kids all night."

After a woman becomes a mother her sex drive can decrease for several reasons. If she has given birth recently, a decrease in estrogen can account for a lack of desire (which is also coincidentally what happens as menopause creeps up). And let's not forget that depletion of energy and God-awful tiredness after a day of keeping up with small children—plus all the other things women do. Menopause, daily schedules, butting heads with your partner are all contributing factors.

In the book *Power Sleep,* we learn that a new parent loses about six hundred hours of sleep in the first year of a baby's life. (Are you starting to see more clearly why sex may be the last thing on your mind?) Post-baby-blues might also contribute, as can a lack of motivation. Who feels like slipping into something more revealing if you are covered with cereal goop and haven't showered in two days?

The vast majority of women I spoke with report that date night usually turns into a family outing. One woman I spoke with, however, had an idea that seems to have sustained through the past nine years and three kids: Her date night is during the week rather than on weekends when so much of life is taken up by family activities. "Sometimes we go out for a quiet, fast dinner and then take a walk; sometimes we play tennis. The only rule is that we cannot talk about the kids unless it is an emergency."

A lack of romantic interest doesn't lie just with new mothers! Many men feel left out of their partner's newfound maternal preoccupation. If the father is feeling sorry for himself during this period, women see their mood as selfish. They then both withdraw even further. Hopefully, as men take more of an increased interest in their small ones (and as more mothers let them), things will continue to improve in this arena.

Unfortunately, this dearth of desire during the early times often becomes habit by the time the child gets older and the daily routine settles in. Here's some good advice to strive for: When you and your partner start to slip away from each other, take some time to remember what attributes you fell in love with in the first place, and what turned you on. Rekindle the romance slowly just as you did in the beginning. Flirt with each other, buy gifts, call to say, "I love you" during the day.

Try whatever you think will work: You and your child's other parent will be together for many years to come.

Life in the Mommy Lane

Following are a few rambling thoughts along the mommy track:

- Children are all given the same script at birth, which include the phrases: "Let me, let me." "Nooooooo." "I didn't get a turn." "But we don't have one in blue." "I didn't make that mess, my hand did." "Please-thankyoumayI." "Mommeeeee!" and my personal favorite, "Mommy will you marry me?" (regardless of gender).

- Your child's script is countered by the one you get: "Good job!" "Use your words." "Would you like a time-out?" "Can you share the trucks (or ball or whatever)?" "If you don't clean up your room, you will lose privileges" and my personal favorite, "Mommy loves you."

- Your mind will rarely be clear and focused exclusively on what you are doing. Even as I am writing this, half my brain is wondering what my son is doing on the other side of the house in the family room.

- If I haven't stressed this enough, let me repeat: Everything you do will take longer. "One day my husband came home from work and couldn't believe I was still in my nightgown. That's because all day my nine-month-old never once let me put her down long enough to get dressed. I had planned to get dressed and clean the kitchen. Somehow, there wasn't any time to do even that!" said a forty-six-year-old new mother.

- We must stop trying to "go go go" from one activity to the next and slow down to our children's level. All things are new to them and not only do they want to know everything (by the way, what are those spindly things on top of the banister called?), they want to share their new findings with you. This is why you wanted a child, remember?

- The average American woman spends only one-seventh of her life either pregnant, nursing or caring for preschool children. If that's the case, many wonder why they rarely get a chance to get dressed by themselves. "I really resent the fact that my husband gets to shower every single day," says a harried forty-two-year-old mother of an eighteen-month-old.

• Like me, you might naively believe your little angel will sleep soundly in his stroller while you have a leisurely lunch in a restaurant with tablecloths. (*Note:* The reason I am so obsessed with dining out is that this activity, coupled with going to the movies, are the two top things women miss most from their former lives.) Do not be tricked.

• Have you ever heard the story about the woman who was able to pick up a car all by herself to rescue her son who was stuck under it? You, too, will find the strength, will and energy to do what you need to do each day then fall into bed exhausted each night, self-satisfied with the great job you are doing and the above-human powers you are developing.

• As your child gets older, your time will be spent (in addition to your other life responsibilities) volunteering in the classroom, driving to and from music lessons, cheering at soccer games, as well as helping with homework. But you'll also start getting more and more "free time" for yourself.

• The reality is there will be days when you wonder what you did besides change diapers on one end and force food into the other, just so you can repeat the whole thing all over again. Remind yourself on those days that, actually, you accomplished a lot. You successfully cared for a totally dependent little being whom you adore. You taught him or her to trust, to feel secure and to be loved. And you got some warm snuggling in as well.

Schedules

The fact that infants sleep and eat a lot might delude you into believing that for the first few months after baby comes home, you will have plenty of time to do things you usually do. The odds are that the second your child comes home, you will see the need for a schedule. Babies respond better to sleeping and eating if they do it at around the same predictable time each day. As your child grows, everyone from your pediatrician to friends who are already grandparents will warn that if you don't get your toddler and preschooler into a regular time for eating, bathing and sleeping, there will be hell to pay later on.

Each child is different, and all children are the same: What this means is that, yes, all families can benefit from a schedule that encompasses the same elements (like those listed above), but not all families should insist on the same timetable. One child may sleep later, another needs more naps, still a third may not nap at all.

Try what works for you first, combined with the recommendations that make sense from other sources, like your child's doctor or your mother-in-law.

Schedules must be open to change. What works this week will not necessarily work once your child is walking, going on playdates, in school, playing football or working on his Ph.D.

Play and Peer Groups

When you are in your forties and all the mothers' groups around you are made up of women in their twenties (this can be especially true if you live in a small community far from a metropolitan area), it can feel quite isolating. You might see yourself as having much more experience in the "real" world than these women and therefore believe you do not have anything in common with them.

Not true. They will also have the interest of their kids at heart; otherwise they wouldn't be taking the time to come to a playgroup. Playgroups are designed not just for the children, but for the mothers to trade war stories and learn from each other. Try to find at least one woman you feel comfortable with.

If you don't know where there is an existing playgroup to join, start a "But I Don't *Feel* Too Old to Be a Mommy!" playgroup of your own. Hang out at the parks to meet other moms. Put a notice in your local parenting publication and read the ones already in there. Check out children's clothing and toy store bulletin boards or ask employees if they know of a group. Stop women who have kids the age of yours at the mall or in the grocery store. Suggest a playdate and exchange phone numbers. Call the maternity ward of your local hospital or ask your adoption agency if they have a newsletter.

Use all those fabulous networking skills you've learned through time.

Outings

Right before we brought Skyler home, I took a hike by myself one morning. I remember thinking, "This is probably the last time I'll be able to get out and do this until he gets married." While that may be a bit of an exaggeration, even simple outings A.C. definitely require planning.

The best rule of thumb to master is that you have to add thirty to forty-five minutes to everything you do. For example, if your shopping excursions include your little one, schedule additional time for getting your child in and out of the car seat; undoing the stroller (then refolding it up once you leave the mall); buckling your little one into the stroller or attaching a baby backpack or sling to yourself (don't forget to put your baby in it); fishing out toys and bottles or sippy cups as well as wipes, pacifier, burp cloths, clean socks and a bib; stashing sweaters, drool-covered toys and assorted sundries. This does not include the time it takes to pick up and restock everything your child pulls off the shelves if he is not in napping mode when you are in the store.

Although this is a lot of extra action on your part, let's consider what it might have been like a few generations ago before women had cars, portable strollers, sippy cups or malls to escape to. Keep that in mind while you are out and about: This perspective raises your outings to the realm of a blessing.

The Bag

Even after your child outgrows the infant stage and you don't have to lug a suitcase full of supplies with you (diapers, wipes, pad, rash cream, cornstarch powder, plastic bags, nursing pads if needed), you will still want to carry "The Bag, Modified." Many smart older mothers who like to have their hands free for hugging and wiping and such, carry a daypack-style "diaper" bag. You can use either a regular daypack or one made specifically for carrying baby's things; these latter usually include a fold-out changing pad. Whichever you choose, make sure it has lots of pockets with zippers. Check out the diaper bag section at the store. You can even find ones with room for a laptop.

Speaking of zippers, those sandwich bags with the zipper-style closures are a mother's best friend: 1) They take up less room than carrying a whole box of something or other. 2) You can tote along just a few Band-Aids at a time rather than the whole container. 3) You can likewise combine a few of this and that into one bag rather than carrying lots of things in lots of bags. 4) The bags are waterproof. 5) Lastly, but of no small importance, the bags are see-through. Buy a variety of sizes and pack with Band-Aids, tissues, wipes, sunblock, waterless hand cleaner, aloe, ipecac syrup, bee sting kit, first aid kit (including antibiotic cream) and any medications you might need.

Other tote-along items: toys, toys, toys and did I mention toys? Restaurant toys (take them out one at a time), travel toys (buy new ones to give out on long trips, again one at a time), pre-inked stamps, stickers, paper (for drawing on rather than the car seat), crayons, markers, bubbles and other one-piece toys are terrific for this purpose. Those over-the-seat organizers are great for keeping a lid on clutter. I use an old gym duffle bag with a zipper to keep everything together on the seat next to my son, so he can grab what he wants. Also, keep sand toys and balls in the car. You never know when you might need to make a quick trip to the park or beach.

Take plenty of snacks along: water, milk or formula at first, then progress to watered-down juice. Buy crackers by the warehouse load; kids can never get enough of them.

Carry a few jars of baby food for infants and raisins, pretzel sticks or cheese sticks as they get older.

Stock the car with a bag of a seasonally appropriate complete changes of clothes for each child: from sweaters in the cooler seasons to watershoes and bathing suits for an impromptu dip during the warmer months. Don't forget the spare socks, hat, mittens and jacket for winter's changing weather.

Include one section in the bag for you: makeup, comb, brush, cell phone, pager, organizer, wallet, phone numbers, etc.

Childcare

In response to so many mothers who work, there is a concerted effort to educate the corporate world about the need for good childcare. A mother's mind is never more focused on her work than when she can feel confident that her children are being cared for in a safe and stimulating environment by nurturing people.

Here's what some mothers told me about childcare:

- "That's my child's life we are talking about. I have to know that he'll be happy when I leave him."

- "I can drop in on her anytime—and I often do. Every time I make a surprise visit, she's involved in story time, singing a song or making a painting. She loves it, and so do I."

- "She gets to do more at day care than I can do with her at home."

Luckily, many companies are realizing what a necessity good childcare is. For instance, Ford Motor Company announced it will open twenty-four-hour childcare facilities in thirty locations.

But you don't have to work away from home in order to have a reason to use childcare. "Even though I don't work outside of the house, I take him a few mornings a week. It works for everyone: He gets time to play with other kids and I get things done I wouldn't be able to otherwise," reports a thirty-seven-year-old mother of a nine-month-old boy.

Sharing in-home childcare is becoming a popular alternative to childcare away from home: You and several other mothers who have a similar child-rearing philosophy can hire a "nanny" to be with your children on a regular basis. This can range from all day to a few days a week to several hours now and then. According to a Northern California childcare resource agency, this is a perfect solution if you are looking for a lower child-to-caregiver ratio. Infants and small children in these situations do very well: They get closer attention and they often have only one or two other children to be with. Where the childcare takes place is open to negotiation: your house? caregiver's house? Discuss with the other family(ies) what kinds of discipline you want, what to do if the caregiver is sick, etc.

Can I Do This?

Even if you've waited, wanted and wished with every fiber of your being for motherhood, once it comes, there will still be times when you wonder, "What made me think I could do this?"

Women have been mothers since time immemorial—and even before that—and have not only survived the rough spots, but thrived.

Even taking into consideration your very normal trepidations, there is no reason to think other than that you will, too.

If It's So Much Work, Why Do It?

Without exception, every mother I heard from had the same unqualified response when I posed that question to her: "Becoming a mother later in life is the best thing I have ever done for myself." Mothers who got started later love every minute of their new lives. They feel enriched beyond how any new job, relationship or place to travel could make them feel:

"I feel so alive."

"The truth is if I haven't been with him all day, I sorely miss him. He can light up any mood."

"I actually feel my body chemistry change when I hold

him to me. Stress falls away, and I am surrounded by light. It feels great."

Is it worth the work? "Life is fuller, richer and deeper beyond my dreams."

That's the simple truth.

CHAPTER 8

Career Considerations After Mommyhood

Q: "Do you work?"

A: "Do you know a mother who doesn't?"

No longer having to choose between parenting or another career—or apologize for their decisions—mothers today take advantage of a variety of career choices available to them. They range from stay-at-home mom to working full time away from home, and from running a small business to configuring a variety of other work combinations.

The Times They Are A-Changing

In contrast to the norm of the 1950s, women no longer expect to cite "housewife" as their lifelong job role, especially since 63 percent with children under age two are in the labor force.

While climbing the corporate ladder seemed to be the prime goal in many women's lives during the 1970s and '80s, shifting attitudes today make us question if having a career should be a woman's most satisfying identity.

Having tried swinging the pendulum in both directions, mothers now want to mix it up; many opt to keep one foot in the labor force even as they are fully entrenched on the home front.

As an enormous number of working mothers force the business world to wake up to the importance of integrating family life with a paying job, career counselor Marty Nemko concludes we are becoming less "work-centric."

Not surprisingly, it's women of our generation who are at the forefront of this quiet revolution—explorers breaking new ground. It's a major lifestyle shift: While workers in past generations spent about 50 percent of their life span in the employment force, most of us will be working well past our halfway mark, into our seventies and beyond. This is especially true when there are children college-age and younger at home.

Finding creative new ways to work (moving the nine-to-five cubicle dweller to home, flextime, job sharing, starting your own business or any combination of these and other options) will help make this shift possible.

Decisions, Decisions, Conflict, Conflict

Having many options available is particularly great news for new older mothers with young children. When motherhood enters your life, your life needs reordering. Your priority becomes what is the most beneficial way to spend your day on behalf of your new child, your whole family, and of course, yourself.

It's a double—nay, *triple*—bind. For all the progress women have made over the last decades, older mothers (indeed, all mothers) remain conflicted over how to spend as much time as needed with family while also having a fulfilling career, whatever form we want that to take.

Your desire to become a mother at this point may very well coincide with a reevaluation of other phases of your life, with your career as a central part of that. Many women at thirty-five and forty have a strong foothold on their career path and a good idea how they want their careers to fit in with the rest of their lives.

But you are rethinking your status quo on more than one level.

Rare is the woman who delays motherhood only to put her child at the bottom of her priority list. Most moms who have waited to have children aren't desirous of a career. While they know a paying job will not fill the void of wanting a child, they know it can fill other voids, most notably those of finances and creativity.

The question becomes, then, how best to mix mothering, the need for an income and desires for career fulfillment with the limitations of time and energy.

For each new older mother, there is a different solution.

What to Consider

When reviewing your options between a career as a full-time stay-at-home mom, starting your own business, working full time or any one of the countless new alternatives, it boils down to a quality-of-life decision. Only you can determine what is the best for your situation.

Determining your financial needs is one way to decide. Start by asking yourself the following questions:

- How much can be cut from the family budget? Would my paycheck be missed? (Most women's incomes provide at least half of the household budget.)
- Can you dip into savings if needed (especially if you've already spent a chunk of it on infertility treatments, adoption or both)?

- Can the family afford to give up your health insurance, paid days off, vacation time, 401k?
- Will the money coming in from your job balance out with the money paid out to childcare and other costs of working (i.e., clothes, commute expense, eating out)?
- Assuming you had the interest, what would be the start-up costs of an at-home business you could run?
- If you go back to work after being out of the business world for several years, will your age then be a factor to consider in finding employment again? Is your chosen industry hard to reenter if you are a woman in your mid-forties or older, especially if you've been out of the loop for a few years? While no one can give you a guarantee about what the next years will bring, talk to your human resources department to see what your chances would be of getting your job back in a few years, months, etc.
- If you choose a full-time stay-at-home career after your child arrives, how will the loss of your income affect you in the long term, not just the short term? Keep in mind that it may be hard to make up for lost income. Do you have savings or investments to fall back on?

These factors are simple enough to figure out with the aid of pencil, paper, calculator or computer; more complex are the factors that can't be tallied along with the bottom line, such as the wear and tear on you. Either end of the job spectrum can cause stress, from staying home full time and missing coworker companionship, to working outside of your home wishing you were at home with your child.

Ask yourself:

- What are your desires, responsibilities, goals?
- What options, alternatives and combinations of resources can you put together to best serve these purposes?
- What kind of support can you expect, especially from your partner or other family members in regard to childcare and/or finances?

Mothering Creates Inventiveness Out of Necessity: New Alternative Ways to Work

When looking at work options these days, anything your fertile mind can conjure up has the possibility of becoming a reality. As a new mother, you may be looking to change the structure and schedule of your present job to accommodate your new status. You are not alone. With half the workforce comprised of women, questions are being raised about deeply entrenched work traditions. The nine-to-five, five-day-work-week-one-size-fits-all conformity that has driven the corporate world is undergoing a shift. One sign is The Work and Family Institute's findings of 1,050 major employers which shows 68 percent offer flexible scheduling, up 17 percent in less than seven years.

Many more companies are jumping on the bandwagon.

A Movement Is Stirring

Companies are beginning to turn their attention from the short term and look to the long term as they learn to become responsive to employees' needs.

Signaling a bright new light on the horizon, a recent survey reports that over two hundred mid-to-large companies now have a work/family manager in the human resources department (some companies have even created work/life committees). Their job is to balance life at work with life at home for the benefit of employees, as well as the company. As one such manager notes, "The days of one work schedule being right for everyone are over with."

Another encouraging survey of 614 employers shows creating flexible schedules is the number-one way in which they hope to retain their employees.

Sequencing

Speaking directly to the point of the working woman's changing needs and showing up smack dab in the middle of the path older mothers find themselves on, *sequencing* has become a new mantra. Coined by author Arlene Rossen

Cardozo in her 1986 book by the same name, sequencing is a catchall phrase for women who want to take time to raise their families but don't want to give up working for the rest of their lives. Maybe they'll take months off from a job, maybe years. Maybe they'll care for their children while also nurturing a part-time job or volunteering their career skills to keep their hand in the action.

Any combination of stay-at-home mom and career outside of the family can be called sequencing, whether you divide your time equally between the two vocations or not. This career shift is accomplished by first finding the best schedule for yourself and your goals and then finding the best place to work this schedule—whether or not it's with your present employer.

The next two sections will help you work it out.

Working Part Time with a Full-Time Life: Getting Your Employer to Change Your Schedule

In a perfect world, you are already working for one of the aforementioned progressive-thinking companies that will easily and cheerfully accommodate your new needs once you become a mother.

If that's not the likely first reaction to your request for a more mommy-friendly schedule from your present employer, here are some things you can do to get your boss to agree to a more flexible work day:

1. Often women who have delayed motherhood have years invested at their job. Therefore their employers are likely to allow more choices, e.g., an extended leave of absence, early retirement, telecommuting (see next page).

2. Another option is to tag team with the child's other parent: the first parent works one week on, one week off, the second parent works opposite weeks (or days or time of day). The pitfalls and positives are obvious: lack of family time all together versus the ongoing presence of one parent at home.

3. If your boss is too hardheaded, you can start now to look for a new job with a better schedule. "Don't be afraid that you are too old to switch careers or get a new degree," advises Rosemary Hartigan, Professor of Management at Antioch University. "Also be aware that many jobs advertised as full time can be negotiated to part time. Don't be intimidated by the ads."

4. If your boss is too hardheaded and you don't want to give up your job, read the next two sections.

New Options for Flexible Schedules Include:

- **Telecommuting** (sometimes called flex-place): Most work is done at home or another location set up with computer, fax, e-mail, etc.

- **Flextime:** Generally, the employee comes to work earlier and leaves earlier, sometimes making up hours with a six-day workweek.

- **Flex Workweek:** More days and shorter hours, or less days and longer hours.

- **Job Sharing:** Two (or more) people share the duties of one job on alternate schedules.

- **Part Time:** Fewer hours or days per week, generally with less equitable pay and benefits.

- **Temporary:** On an as-needed basis, the employee will most likely be working at different offices, jobs, hours, days.

- **Contract Labor and Consultation,** which are also options, generally fall more under the heading of running your own business (see page 121).

See the Resources section of this book for support organizations to contact.

Getting Your Boss to Agree

Once you decide what kind of schedule you want, put it into the form of a proposal and present it to your employer. Experts say the following benefits should be included in your proposal:

- **Clearly define your goals.** Have them clearly defined in your own mind first. Do you want to be home by nap time every afternoon, come into the office only once a week, put in no more than twenty hours each week?

- **Play up your loyalty and track record with the company.** Advise management that you will continue with the same fine caliber of work whether you are in the office or working from home.

- **Overcome objections** before they are presented to you. For instance, your boss might ask how he or she can monitor your work. Assure him or her that you will check in frequently through phone, fax, e-mail, etc.

- **Point out that the new schedule will benefit** your company, not just you and your family. Will they save on company-paid benefits?

- **Suggest a trial period.** All new jobs have a trial period anyway, whether or not it is in writing. This will reinforce your serious intent.

- **Ask for prorated benefits.** There is a good chance you

won't get any, so reserve this as a negotiating point.

- **Detail how you will cover sick days,** vacation time or other days off.

- **If anyone else at your company** (or with similar positions at other companies) is working the way you are proposing, describe how well it is going. Get recommendations from their bosses.

- **Let your employer know that employees who telecommute** are often more productive away from the distractions of coworkers. Your company is likely to get more work out of you in less time with less absenteeism.

- **Lastly, don't give up.** If you are turned down on any of your points—or on the whole proposal—try again in a few months.

"When I tell people what my schedule is," a forty-four-year-old mother of one-year-old twins says, "they tell me how lucky I am. But I created this. It took a lot of convincing on my part to get my boss to agree to let me work two-and-a-half days out of my house and only one and a half days in the office."

"Sure I'm making less money now," says another midlife mother, who converted her high-pressure full-time legal secretarial job into a job share, "but it was an easy decision for me to make once I realized how much I wanted to be home with my child."

The Changing Workforce

"If companies are expected to survive," says workplace researcher Judy Rosener, "they have to be open to all segments of the changing workforce."

Broaching your boss with new options for your work schedule can feel intimidating because you are one of the pioneers breaking down old ways to work. If it seems overwhelming, remember that it wasn't so long ago that becoming a mother at your age was also pretty much unheard of.

Telecommuting

Whether it's full or part time, doing some of your work at home instead of full time in the office carries with it lots of obvious benefits (number one being that you are home with your children), as well as responsibilities.

Survey after survey shows that work-at-home telecommuting moms are more productive than they are in the office. Despite this, bosses and co-workers are often suspicious that the telecommuting employee has it "too easy." As a result, extra work may be loaded onto her, along with high expectations that she will always be available to answer the telephone, fax or e-mail upon demand. To allay these fears—at least at the beginning of your telecommuting arrangement—it is advisable to have "face time" at the office. Showing up at the start or end of the business day will demonstrate that you are on the same schedule as everyone else.

The reality is that far from spending time on the couch with a remote control in one hand and an iced tea in the other, a telecommuter—like full-time stay-at-home moms or those running their own business—can work a lot longer than the prescribed eight hours per day, especially as she also cares for her kids.

Happily though, as a telecommuting mom, you can also take time for an occasional impromptu trip to the ice cream store with the newest object of your affection.

Opting for a Full-Time Career Away from Home

A recent survey may have shocked some people, but for many full-time working moms it was no surprise. The survey showed that many working parents actually look forward to "escaping" to their full-time jobs away from home.

This survey is not a denigration of how parents enjoy and love their children; the reasons for having a full-time job can be many. One often-stated reason—aside from the most evident, income—is the camaraderie.

Women who become stay-at-home moms, on the coattails of working with people who often become as close as family, can feel lonely, isolated, "out of the loop" as well as unchallenged, unstimulated and devoid of creativity once they stay home, particularly at the beginning.

This is reinforced up by a Cornell University study that interviewed 745 women; the study found that mothers who left full-time jobs to become stay-at-home moms were more distressed than mothers who stayed on the job after the arrival of their child.

For older mothers, this is not necessarily so. The urge to be a stay-at-home mom is most often overwhelming. The decision to go back to work when there is a new child at home is a very hard one to make; this is especially so for women who have waited. Even if she has a full-time job outside of the house, a new mother's newest career—motherhood—supercedes all others in her heart.

No matter what else she does, or where she physically spends her day, a mother is always a mother; even if she works outside of the house. She is never just a "part-time" mom. Full-time working moms of every age confide they spend a lot of time thinking about their children while they are on the job. "I don't give my all to my job as I once did," confessed one midlife mom.

Because of her dual role—and no matter how much she needs and likes her job—the working mom's laments strike: ambivalence, worry, guilt, sacrifice, little personal time, being pulled from all directions, waning energy.

These are the words used by full-time working moms to describe their lifestyle . . . unless they learn how to manage the accompanying chronic stress.

Easing the Stress

Another survey produced a collective sigh of relief from working moms. It shows that children who are in good, nurturing and caring day care fare on a par with children with stay-at-home moms.

If you'll be working at a job other than motherhood, finding quality childcare should be foremost in your plans. Consistent care should be a priority. Children do better when they know what they can expect each day; that includes familiar faces. Start checking out places now. Some of the very best might have a waiting list, so it can never be too soon. Also, read the "Reality Bites" chapter of this book for more about day care.

A possible adverse result of having your child in group day care is they become more exposed to every sniffle—and worse—that's going around. And if you are rundown from everything you are trying to juggle, there's a chance you'll also get sick. Who, then, will care for the kids?

One strategy for heading off stress is to plan ahead for those eventual sick days (yours and your child's) by creating plans ahead of time. Try trading for a night out with a stay-at-home mom or contracting with a drop-in day care that specializes in sick children. A plan should also be in place for finding an emergency backup if your child needs an adult on the scene in the middle of a busy day: Do you have relatives nearby who can handle such rare problems for you?

Is there a mother's club you can join that offers such services? If not, start one (again, check out "Reality Bites").

In yet another survey, surprising no one this time, the Families and Work Institute found that mothers with a full-time job outside of the home are more likely to sacrifice their own personal time in favor of family or job. For instance, full-time working moms often feel like they have to wait on their children as soon as they get home to "make up" for lost time, ignoring their own quiet-time needs.

Many books are written on how women can take care of themselves and the importance of having personal, quiet time. Buy yourself one of these books, follow the ideas in it and treasure it. Having personal time is core to sanity.

While you may put yourself at the bottom of your to-do list, your family doesn't.

If you collapse, it helps no one.

Starting a Home-Based Business

Mention the possibility of running a home-based business to mothers—new and seasoned alike—and watch their eyes glaze over, their mouths fashion into sappy grins. This vision of sugarplums has convinced ten million mothers, so far, to open the door on their own home-based business—even if that door only leads to the kitchen table.

You can make it ten million and one.

No longer just a stop-gap measure until mothers can get a "real" job, Clifford Holtz of AT&T's small business wing says that "Momprenuers are the single fastest-growing type of business out there."

For many older mothers, this comes as close to mommy nirvana as any woman can hope for.

Trade-Offs

Running a business from the house while mothering young children doesn't exactly equal a day at the beach, even if your former co-workers might think so. In addition to the usual run of challenges in starting a business, you have your child's needs directly under your nose (while reminding yourself that this is also the big plus to working at home).

While on the face of things a home-based business can look like the best option, there are drawbacks . . . well, actually there are trade-offs; but life is a series of trade-offs, isn't it?

For starters, you will not be able to slip out for a quick bite without a lot of pre-planning. You will also be the busiest woman on the block. "I had taken my son to his music lesson and planned to sit in the waiting room to catch up on some work while he was in his lesson. But when I got there, I realized I forgot my laptop. It would take too long to run home and get it. I had nothing to do but sit. It felt kind of funny. I had forgotten what it was like with nothing to do," recalls one forty-one-year-old momprenuer with two kids under five years of age. Remaining focused is a super challenge when the kids are home sick or when they are bored and want you to help them build a rocket ship—again (which is what's going on in my house as I attempt to write these words).

You won't always be able to choose your work hours, but you can be there when your child is sick, needs a hug or wants to give one.

You will also trade for time off: You may work late one night so that you can escort your child to a birthday party the next morning. Juggling motherhood, career, family and other personal interests can be tricky; whatever you can do to diminish stress is a blessing. Being able to control your schedule is one big way to lower stress.

While the needs of both your child and your business constantly change, there will be days when you wonder why you didn't do this sooner.

The biggest complaints of home-based entrepreneurs (as well as stay-at-home moms) stem from the days when isolation and loneliness weigh heavy. Those times are compounded when you haven't changed out of the same fleece pants and fluffy slippers days in a row, remaining indoors incommunicado, a coughing baby in the next room.

This is why your house comes with a door: Use it! Go outside. Go to lunch, go to playgroup—just go! A change of scenery is a marvelous curative.

Perhaps the biggest trade-off comes in the form of less income, especially if you are starting a business from scratch in a field new to you. But as your child spends more time away from home in school, more time is put into the business leading to larger earnings later on.

'Tis Wonderful

The advantages of running your own business from home are obvious. Having dominance over your schedule *plus* being around to watch your child develop every day or help out in her classroom is pretty wonderful.

A less obvious advantage is the role model you will be creating for your children: With you at work in the next room, your children will get a much better idea of what's involved in being committed to a task than if you were off somewhere called "at work." They will witness you reaping the fruits of your labor, learning firsthand what's involved in earning an income.

Your children may even be able to help; even preschoolers can offer an opinion on your package design, put stamps on envelopes for a mailing and keep quiet while Mommy makes an important phone call.

Gearing Up

What do you need to make the transition from working outside of your home for someone else to running your own home-based business? One thing it takes is knowing yourself: Generally the older a woman gets, the more she follows her inner voice, gaining more insight with each passing year, no longer following the crowd for fear of missing out.

Not so sure you can keep head and motivation together to run your own home-based business? Check out the qualities you may need to gear up:

- Can you flow from one task to another relatively easily—from phone call to making breakfast to supervising a finger painting to following up on a fax?
- What about unexpected interruptions to your perfectly planned routine? Can you identify and act on fluctuating priorities? Flexibility is a major key to being a happy entrepreneur.
- Do you respect your own schedule? If you do not respect the hours you've set up to work, no one else will. Family, friends and others will take their cue from you. Letting people know politely, but firmly, that yes, you are at home, but you are working, will establish your credibility.
- While it is not totally impossible to run a home business without any childcare for your young ones, it is

close to impossible. If you don't want to use outside day care, hire a teenager to read and play with your child while you work. It gives both you and your child a break.

- Are you organized? If not, treat yourself to a professional organizer. It will give you more time with your family and your business and pays for itself in the end.
- Are you self-disciplined? Can you assign yourself a working time frame along with goals and then accomplish what you want without getting distracted?
- Are you self-motivated? Are you willing to practice self-motivating techniques?
- If you are stuck for ideas, see a career counselor. Seventy percent of mothers who start a home-based business turn a former career into a niche. This is an opportunity to do what you've always wanted to do rather than what you've always done.
- If you are pregnant or going through an adoption or infertility process, take this time to plan ahead.
- Keep a sense of humor.

Staying Organized

Your business cards and letterhead are printed, the fax machine is installed and a few clients are even making their way to you. You are proud of yourself, juggling a growing business with a growing child.

If you have any one thing to thank for this success, it would have to be organization. Without it, you'd feel more like a circus act than a businesswoman. A few hints:

- Learn to say no. Saying yes to a fun midday excursion to the zoo when faced with a day of balancing numbers is tempting; but if it doesn't serve your immediate goals, just say "No."
- If you cannot stop what you are doing to color with your toddler, tell him or her when you can and then follow through.
- Take time for yourself to segue between work and home life. A short breather, say the length of a brief commute, will go a long way toward shaking off your work mode and slipping into your mommy mode.
- Make a schedule and stick with it as closely as possible.
- Your time is limited. Use as many worthy shortcuts as you can. For instance, bulk-up work-related errands, and do those run-around chores once, not all day.
- Don't work on family time. Write family events and work-related appointments in two different colors on your calendar.
- Create a hands-off boundary around your work space— even if it's just a corner of the family computer desk.
- Always keep in mind why you are doing this.

Full-Time Stay-at-Home Mom

"They are only young once—and it goes fast. I want to be right there, experiencing every day with my son," says a forty-one-year-old new mother. Many older mothers agree; they say they haven't waited to become mothers (or to mother again) to do anything else except relish their role full time. "I won't lie and say that there aren't days that I don't miss my old job, but being with my family—there's never a comparison."

"This is hard work," says another mom who is home full time. "It's much tougher being a stay-at-home mother than anyone can imagine."

As mothers, we are the Chief Operating Officers in guiding the shape of our children's lifelong behaviors, beliefs, feelings, skills and interests. It's a job description with lots of creative challenges and fulfillment.

It is nonsense to suggest that an older mother's decision to stay home has anything to do with a fear that she can't hold down a "real" job. Stay-at-home mothering isn't for wimps.

Blessedly, we have moved past the perceptions of the 1970s that looked down at stay-at-home moms, or worse, the 1950s when stay-at-home moms were referred to as "housewives," conjuring up an image of being wed to the oven. Today, parenting is enjoying a renewed respect; moms who stay home with their children full-time are supported and admired, even envied.

The Toughest Job You'll Ever Love

Stay-at-home moms work hard and get little recognition from the outside. They get no paycheck, no paid sick or vacation days, few awards and fewer days off. They don't qualify for workmen's comp, disability or unemployment insurance when their full-time job grows up and starts school. A stay-at-home mom makes sacrifices for her job just like any other working mom, including big changes in lifestyle —especially if she is used to working outside of the home. More often than not, she also has to keep a close watch on the purse strings: "I love being a stay-at-home mom. I hate worrying about money," one mother of two little ones says.

And to top it off, she's working for someone who can't even speak yet!

As an accomplished woman with educational, career and life experiences, you might wonder what life will be like diapering, feeding, reading and singing the same song verses repeatedly, especially if you've had years of a freer lifestyle and adult-oriented schedule.

The shift to full-time mommyhood—especially later in life can be slightly unnerving if your identity has been wrapped up in a career. The 1996 June/July issue of *Population Today* magazine found "there is a difference in what women expect their careers in motherhood to be and what it really is, even with lots of forethought." The magazine also found that women who delay motherhood may have problems giving up the control they have been used to in their relationships and careers.

Staying at home to be a full-time mother can be very stressful, especially if you are a first-time older mother with an infant or toddler. "It's my experience that a stay-at-home mom is rarely actually staying at home. We are always off doing things," says one forty-one-year-old mother of three children under five.

Isolation and boredom can be factors; finding other mothers with whom to form a playgroup can help. Even if you don't become close buddies with these other women, it is good to be able to trade war stories, learn from each other, mingle while the children socialize and realize that you are not alone.

Take advantage of nap times or times when your child plays by himself or herself to do something for just you; on days when these breaks aren't forthcoming, throw up your hands and give thanks for the opportunity you have been given to be a mother at this point in your life.

When it comes to housework, try to stay focused on your primary job description: the care and feeding of your child. On the days when you can't get anything done because your baby won't let you put him or her down long enough to pull on a pair of skivvies, let alone vacuum, cook and shop, remind yourself of this.

So, you may be wondering, what's in it for me? Simple. You will be there every step of the way. What a payoff!

The Slaying of the Super Mom

No matter which career you choose—stay-at-home mom, working full time, or anything in between—you can't do it all. Along with dumping antiquated and limiting images of what mothers should and shouldn't be, we are gratefully dumping the image that women can and should do it all.

The Super Mom figure led mothers to believe they must rise to the top of their careers, oversee growing children while combining the skills of a goddess, Julia Child and the diva Madonna—and not confusing in which room each skill is to be used. And all the while, never losing it.

It's an image that's been impossible to live up to. Believing there was something wrong with them when they couldn't do it all, many mothers suffered unnecessary guilt trying to live up to what the media portrayed as the ideal.

You may want it all, but having it all at once is challenging, at best. It's humanly impossible to be responsible for everything all the time. Thankfully, the myth of the Super Mom is finally getting an overdue burial.

Strategies for All Moms

"Men work from sun to sun, but a woman's work is never done." Unfortunately, current research shows this little ditty still rings true. Mothers work a full fifteen hours per week more than fathers; they are still doing the bulk of the housework. Mothers who have careers in addition to motherhood are especially hard hit: 46 percent of them say they worry constantly about balancing the demands of family and work.

Formulating tactics for your new role keeps a lid on the worry. The following strategies are applicable to all mothering/ career combos:

- Schedule breaks for yourself and use them. From a minimum twenty minutes to put your feet up with a cup of tea to an evening spent by yourself at the bookstore, never ignore your own time off. Without these breaks, you cannot keep your own inner resources intact, and without that, you will not function at your highest.

- Hire baby-sitters on a regular basis. Go on dates with your partner to keep your relationship thriving.

- Keep the telephone number of at least one stay-at-home mom or nearby relative with you at all times to call in the event your child needs to be picked up from childcare or school when you are not able to do so.

- Go high-tech. Get a cell phone and/or pager so you can keep in touch with the parent or sitter at home; a cell phone is also good in the event the car breaks down when you are out with your child.

- Set a schedule and stick with it as best you can without

driving yourself crazy. What are the priorities for the week? Try not to tackle more than three things at any one time.

Daddies Are Parents, Too

Most men today are more involved in the raising of their children than their fathers were; daddies today are hands-on when it comes to changing diapers, taking kids to the playground and reading stories at bedtime. But while things are shifting, they are still not equitable. One way you can help make it more so is to clue Daddy in. Make your child's other parent aware of every nuance of your child's life, so that he can be more involved. If your child has started to shift nap schedules, went down the big slide today or has his first dentist appointment tomorrow, don't keep it a secret.

Also, don't seize all the responsibility away from your partner. This is true even if you choose to be a stay-at-home mom. It is both of your responsibility to see that your child gets a bedtime story. Dad will probably jump at the chance to be more involved.

Another option for working out the career/mommyhood thing is Daddy staying at home full time. Albeit still more rare than stay-at-home moms, dads at home are not an unheard of phenomenon any longer. Have you discussed this option with your partner yet?

And Finally . . .

As women who long for motherhood, we can agree that raising our children is central in importance to us. However, we are not stamped from cookie-cutter molds; our needs and lifestyles vary.

Let us respect and rejoice in each other's career decisions. Let us not be judgmental; instead, let us cheer each other on as someone who is just like us—later-in-life mothers.

6757058862

READER/CUSTOMER CARE SURVEY

We care about your opinions. Please take a moment to fill out this Reader Survey card and mail it back to us.
As a special **"thank you"** we'll send you exciting news about interesting books and a valuable **Gift Certificate**

Please PRINT using ALL CAPITALS

Name
First _____ MI.□ Last Name _____

Address _____

City _____ ST □□ Zip _____

Phone # (□□□) □□□ - □□□□   Fax # (□□□) □□□ - □□□□

Email _____

(1) Gender:
○ Female
○ Male

(2) Age:
○ 13-19   ○ 40-49
○ 20-29   ○ 50-59
○ 30-39   ○ 60+

(3) Your children's age(s):
Please fill in all that apply.
○ 6 or Under   ○ 15-18
○ 7-10   ○ 19+
○ 11-14

(8) Marital Status:
○ Married
○ Single
○ Divorced / Widowed

(9) W as this book:
○ Purchased For Yourself?
○ Received As a Gift?

(10)How many HCI books have you bought or read?
○ 1   ○ 3
○ 2   ○ 4+

(11) Did this book meet your expectations?
○ Yes
○ No

(12) How did you find out about this book? *Please fill in ONE.*
○ Personal Recommendation
○ Store Display
○ TV/Radio Program
○ Bestseller List
○ Website
○ Advertisement/Article or Book
○ Catalog or Mailing
○ Other _____

(13) What FIVE subject areas do you enjoy reading about most? *Rank only FIVE.*
Choose 1 for your favorite, 2 for second favorite, etc.

	1	2	3	4	5
Self Development	○	○	○	○	○
Parenting	○	○	○	○	○
Spirituality/Inspiration	○	○	○	○	○
Family and Relationships	○	○	○	○	○
Health and Nutrition	○	○	○	○	○
Recovery	○	○	○	○	○
Business/Professional	○	○	○	○	○
Entertainment	○	○	○	○	○
Sports	○	○	○	○	○
Teen Issues	○	○	○	○	○
Pets	○	○	○	○	○

BA1

TAPE IN MIDDLE; DO NOT STAPLE

BUSINESS REPLY MAIL
FIRST-CLASS MAIL PERMIT NO 45 DEERFIELD BEACH, FL

POSTAGE WILL BE PAID BY ADDRESSEE

HEALTH COMMUNICATIONS, INC.
3201 SW 15TH STREET
DEERFIELD BEACH FL 33442-9875

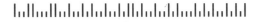

FOLD HERE

BA1

9396058864

(25) Are you:
O A Parent?
O A Grandparent

(18) Where do you purchase most of your books?
Please fill in your top TWO choices only.
O General Bookstore
O Religious Bookstore
O Warehouse / Price Club
O Discount or Other Retail Store
O Website
O Book Club / Mail Order

(20) What type(s) of magazines do you SUBSCRIBE to?
Fill in up to FIVE categories.
O Parenting
O Sports
O Fashion
O Business / Professional
O World News / Current Events
O General Entertainment
O Homemaking, Cooking, Crafts
O Women's Issues
O Other (please specify) _____

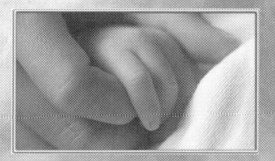

PART THREE

Getting to Mommyhood

CHAPTER 9

The Preconception Checkup: Taking Care of Yourself *Before* You Try to Get Pregnant

T rying to conceive once you are past thirty-five can be an all-consuming proposition, especially when you are having a problem with infertility. Undergoing often-arduous fertility treatments can mean other considerations get put on the back burner. By the time you finally do get pregnant, some problems that got overlooked in the process might be difficult to correct.

That's where the *pre*conception exam comes in. It is the step to take *before* you try to get pregnant.

If you are thinking about becoming pregnant (or if you are already trying), your first order of business should be a preconception checkup. This is also true for your husband.

The logic of undergoing such an exam couldn't be more obvious: First of all, a preconception checkup will ensure that you are sowing the seeds for a healthy pregnancy. Second, while it is wise to be forearmed with knowledge when undertaking something of this magnitude (a new life), it is also cost-effective: Fixing health concerns before the baby becomes a reality saves wear and tear on the wallet, as well as the nerves.

Become Your Doctor's Partner

Health care is a partnership between the health-care provider and the patient. It is the patient's responsibility to supply the health-care provider all the information she can in order for the doctor to do his or her job to the best of his or her ability. Too, an informed patient is the best kind, since she is more likely to reach better decisions. She makes an enormous contribution to a positive outcome for her pregnancy, labor, delivery and health of her baby.

Prevention is the ultimate key to good health. A preconception checkup is one of the best prevention tools. Once a woman is pregnant, the chance to correct many problems becomes lost to her; the sooner she can be seen, the sooner concerns can be identified and fixed.

A Healthy Woman Is Likely to Have Healthy Babies

The Preconception Visit

Too many obstetricians segregate pregnancy and prenatal care from delivery and postpartum care. The new thinking in the field of obstetrics, however, is to integrate all aspects of childbirth.

For women beyond thirty-five and forty, this pregnancy may be the last (or only) shot at carrying a baby full term into a healthy life, while remaining in good health themselves. These dual goals make the preconception visit particularly critical for the older mother.

A preconception visit not only looks at risks, it also advises women on what constitutes health during this period of her life. The exam results in lower infant mortality rates as well as boosting the odds for maternal health.

Some Facts

Age unto itself is not the major concern it once was for midlife pregnancies. This is because most pregnancies of older mothers turn out to be low risk, according to Dr. Roger Lemke, the Director of Maternal Fetal Medicine at the St. Vincent Family Life Center. It is the natural course that the aging process follows that is the concern: Thyroid problems, diabetes, even asthma can all increase with age. Therefore, women who get pregnant at a later age are at risk because of their age and preexisting health complaints.

In 1989, the U.S. Department of Health and Human Services conducted a symposium at which they presented findings on the importance of prenatal care. In "A Report of the Public Health Service Expert Panel on the Content of Prenatal Care," the agency found:

- "The most important doctor visit of all happens before a woman becomes pregnant."

- Over 25 percent of women thirty-five and over have preexisting conditions that could affect their pregnancy. Over age forty, that number increases to 27.2 percent.

- Most women have six or seven concerns—such as genetic testing—they should correct or be informed about prior to getting pregnant.

- A woman who undergoes a preconception checkup demonstrates seriousness in her attention to her health. Doctors find that these women are more likely to follow a healthy regimen once they do get pregnant.

- If problems do exist, they can be treated without any potential harm to the fetus before conception.

What Should Your Preconception Exam Cover?

"A preconception visit differs from a regular doctor or ob/gyn visit in that it focuses on integrating medical, psychological and social data with its potential impact on future pregnancy," concludes panel member Dr. Irwin R. Merkatz. Once the results are known, action can be taken. "Women make changes for a baby that they wouldn't make otherwise," notes Merkatz.

Doctors also find that women who have undergone a preconception exam are more relaxed during their pregnancies.

Following are listings of what every preconception exam should cover. The chances are you will not have problems in many—indeed, most—of these areas. However, you will want to screen for as many areas as make sense for you and your doctor.

Genetic Screenings

Screening for genetic problems is one of the main reasons for a preconception examination. It will determine the risk factor for certain more troublesome birth defects prior to conception. A personal and family history fills in the picture—including environmental factors at work and home.

Here are some genetic concerns that can be tested for prior to pregnancy. The ethnic group each disease is known to be prevalent in is also listed. If your heritage includes any of these groups, you should be tested.

1. **Tay-Sachs:** Eastern Europeans and Ashkenazi Jews.

2. **Thalassemia:** Italians and other descendants of Mediterranean heritage.

3. **Sickle-Cell Anemia:** African heritage.

Genetics testing may also rule out cystic fibrosis, nuerophilia and even recurring pregnancy loss.

Other Tests for Women Beyond Thirty-Five and Over Forty

Patients should request that blood testing and other screenings usually performed after pregnancy be tested now if they have not been done recently. These include screenings for anemia, blood type, toxoplasmosis, Pap smear, mammogram, HIV, urinalysis, herpes, risk assessment for spontaneous abortion, hepatitis, immunity to rubella (if you are not immune, get an immunization shot right away; once you are pregnant, you will not be able to get immunized).

Questions Your Doctor Should Ask You

Your doctor should be informed about all special concerns or conditions you have. Include in these any infections, ovarian cysts, worrisome Pap smears, endometriosis, fibroids; also, any medications you may be taking as well as vitamins. Inform your doctor about the type of diet you eat, if you've had any past miscarriages, abortions or stillbirths, as well as venereal diseases. Your doctor should also ask about your general health and the health of your family members, high blood pressure, heart conditions, epilepsy, lung, liver or kidney disorders.

Your doctor will also need to know about any family or personal incidence of mental retardation, cerebral palsy, muscular dystrophy, cystic fibrosis, hemophilia, spina bifida and other serious conditions. Some are genetically inheritable; others increase the risk of occurrence.

Inform your doctor about your environment at work as well as at home. Do you work with any chemicals? Are you in front of a computer screen all day? Is your home brand new? Do you have an older home that might contain asbestos in the ceiling?

To be certain of your living environment, you might want to hire an environmental expert to check your home for possible pockets of concern.

You can then make any changes you might deem necessary. This will not only make the environment healthier for your pregnancy, but also for your baby once he or she comes home.

The food you ingest as you get close to becoming pregnant is now recognized to be a very important factor;

inform your doctor not only about what you eat, but how you eat, e.g., do you skip meals, do you always eat three squares a day, are you a vegetarian or on a special diet?

If you start a new medication during this time—or especially after you become pregnant—inform your doctor immediately.

Who Should Provide the Exam?

A variety of health-care providers can provide you with your preconception exam, including:

- primary physician
- obstetrician
- nurse-midwife
- pre-pregnancy clinic
- genetic counselor
- fertility specialist

It is also beneficial to talk with a psychotherapist about possible emotional factors that exist or that might crop up, such as handling the loss of fertility and the role stress plays on pregnancy.

The Daddy Factor

While the woman carries the baby, she does not get pregnant alone. Therefore, the health of your baby's father should also be checked prior to conception. Getting pregnant is not a female responsibility alone; it is a partnership physically, emotionally and spiritually.

A similar thorough examination of his medical history and lifestyle should be undertaken. His home environment (if different from yours), as well as work environment should likewise be considered.

Men are infertile in equal numbers to women; however, if the couple's infertility is a sperm issue, it can be identified and fixed with much greater ease than if the fertility problem is the woman's. For this reason alone, your partner's sperm should be checked for health, motility, etc., prior to pregnancy attempts.

Men are warned not to smoke or overuse alcohol while trying to get their wife pregnant. Smoking can damage sperm, as can a lack of antioxidants in the diet, especially vitamins C and E. Smoking also lowers the sperm count.

It is also helpful to have your partner on the same nutritional path as you are during this time. Aside from the obvious benefits of increased health for him as well as the baby, if you are both eating well, you won't be resentful while you're on a steady diet of tofu and rice cakes as he's popping beers and throwing chips down his throat.

Start Caring for Yourself Right Now

Even if you count yourself in the undecided column when it comes to getting pregnant, caring for yourself in the ways suggested here will only serve to make your life better no matter if you go through childbirth, adoption or lifelong childlessness. Ancient Tibetan wisdom says that parental choices attract the child who will incarnate and so influence the nature and quality of the child who enters a family. Extrapolated into Western philosophy, consciously caring for yourself will give you and your child the healthiest chances.

If you are trying to get pregnant but you haven't been successful, you may be lulled (falsely) into the belief that you can put your feet up with a nightly glass of wine and a smoldering cigarette. Picture this: In a few weeks you find out you have been pregnant before you knew about it. Is worrying whether or not that nightly glass of wine could have harmed your fetus worth the drink? Probably not.

The period when you are trying to conceive is also a good time to gain or lose weight if needed. Women who are too thin can be at a health risk when pregnant just as women who are overweight. Women who are too thin have a tendency to give birth to low-weight babies and a possible succession of a host of other problems. Overweight women, for example, can experience edema, which swells ankles, feet and hands.

Stop smoking (if you do smoke) and insist that your partner do likewise. Not only is secondhand smoke harmful to you and your fetus, it can harm your partner's sperm.

Pursue a basic smart living lifestyle that embodies:

- **Exercise:** Check with your doctor about how much and what kind of exercise is good for you now, as well as after you become pregnant.

- **Nutrition:** Knowledgeable obstetricians fully agree that the nutritional health of the mother prior to getting pregnant can make the difference. Check to make sure your diet includes plenty of folic acid, a B vitamin. If this important ingredient is missing from your diet, your baby could wind up with neural tube defects such as spina bifida. Read more about nutrition in the "Pregnancy" and "In It for the Long Haul" chapters of this book.

- **Start taking prenatal vitamins.** Prenatal vitamins contain the same ingredients and often in the same degree (sometimes even less) than many over-the-counter vitamins you might already be taking. Check with your doctor and then talk to a reliable dietician, nutritionist and health food store vitamin buyer.

- **Environmental changes:** Do you work or live in an environment that might be unhealthy for you and your fetus? Hire an expert to examine your surroundings at home; if feasible, ask your boss to do so at work and then make the changes necessary.

• **Make an appointment** with a health-care provider for yourself and your partner today. Your baby will thank you.

CHAPTER 10

Infertility and the New Technology: Here's What You Need to Know Now

If you are over thirty-five or more than forty and having difficulty getting pregnant, or if you know someone who is "trying to conceive" (on one Web site they refer to themselves as "TTCs"), you understand the meaning of the word *obsession*. A whole new world, a whole new language opens up for TTCs; decisions are to be made at every turn: "Should I undergo another cycle of IVF?" "How much longer am I going to subject myself, my husband and our bank account to this?" "Should I start looking into adoption?"

Having spent most of her adult life trying to *avoid* pregnancy, it is frustrating—indeed, devastating—when a woman who is at last ready (read *anxious!*) to get pregnant, can't. When dealing with a biological clock, the saying, "It's never too late" doesn't apply. Women in this age group are often quite flustered to find out that they can't get pregnant just because they want to.

The American Society for Reproductive Medicine reports that for women under thirty there is a 20 percent chance of getting pregnant in any given month. The odds drop to 5 percent by the time a woman reaches forty. It is evident that time is of the essence. Therefore, unlike women in their twenties or early thirties, an older woman should seek the help of a fertility specialist as soon as possible if she is having trouble getting pregnant.

Add to this mix the news that men also have a biological clock—and its alarm goes off much earlier than a woman's. According to the Journal of Human Reproduction, once a man passes age twenty-four, the older he is the harder it is to get his partner pregnant, *regardless of her age.*

This news flash bursts the bubble on another myth: Infertility is not strictly the woman's "fault." As a matter of fact, it affects men and women in equal numbers. Each sex suffers a 35 percent rate of infertility; another 20 percent is blamed on problems unique to the couple. The remaining 10 percent is a result of unknown causes.

Infertility affects about ten million people at any one time. Described on network television as a "horrible disease that's not well-treated by our government," the percentage of women who delay childbearing suffer infertility in the highest numbers:

Fertility drops 30 to 40 percent in the mid-thirties to mid-forties; at age fifty, it becomes almost zero.

The good news is that if there is such a thing as an opportune time to be infertile, it is now. The prospects get better all the time. Today the acronym ART (assisted reproductive technologies) has become a household word, at least in households where the alarms on biological clocks are chiming. While there are no guarantees in the fertility game—only about one out of five couples attempting ART actually wind up with a baby—the last few years have played witness to the birth of remarkable new technologies which raise the stakes, offering encouraging odds even to women already in menopause.

As one forty-nine-year-old prospective mother says, "Hey, the technology is there, and there's no reason not to go for it."

We've Truly Come a Long Way, Er, Baby

Not only is ART improving each day, but our attitudes about "older mothers" are also undergoing a positive metamorphosis. It wasn't that long ago that doctors earmarked the folders of first-time pregnant women over thirty-five as "elderly primigravida," a wholly derogatory term rarely seen any longer (*Note:* If your ob/gyn marks *your* folder with this term, run). Just a few generations ago, babies born to women in their early thirties were known as "change-of-life" babies.

While it appears that bearing children at our ages is an anomaly, we are in reality only returning to what the norm was at the turn of the last century: Women bore children into their late thirties and forties up until the 1950s (albeit not usually with first babies, as is the case today). Younger women started staying home—the war was over, the economy was healthy—and they started raising babies.

While we may be returning to a time when women give birth later in life, the face of how we get there has changed forever. With assisted reproduction technology, there can be as many as five people involved in producing the birth of a baby: egg donor, sperm donor, gestational mother, contracting mother and contracting father.

Dr. Rick Paulson predicts (he's the fertility specialist who aided the world's oldest mother at sixty-three in getting pregnant), "Women will have the capability of getting pregnant one day as long as they live." A report in the *Los Angeles Times* lets us see the beginning of that prediction: 50 percent of women fifty to fifty-four are theoretically fertile.

Commenting on Paulson's famous patient, TV commentator Jane Pauley summed up: "She is one of the world's oldest known women to give birth as of now, but she won't be alone soon."

How Conception Occurs

Without *every one* of these steps, pregnancy cannot occur:

1. Healthy eggs are produced from the ovaries.

2. The fallopian tubes must be unblocked in order for the egg to go through it where it meets the . . .

3. Healthy sperm merges with one or more healthy eggs in the fallopian tubes.

4. The lining of the uterus is prepared (that's progesterone's job), so that the fertilized egg can be "implanted" (attaching itself successfully to the lining of the uterus).

5. Then the right hormones are needed to nourish the fertilized, implanted egg.

If That's All There Is to It, Why Aren't You Pregnant Yet?

The Most Common Causes of Women's Infertility

- **Delaying childbearing:** Delaying motherhood in and of itself is the single biggest cause of infertility in women past thirty-five. Women are born with all the eggs they will ever have—about two million—as opposed to men, who produce about seventy-two million new sperm each day. Good fertile eggs run out about five to ten years before the onset of menopause, explains Dr. Eldon Schriock, former director of the fertility program at the University of California, San Francisco, and present director of the San Francisco Fertility Center. If menopause occurs at about age fifty-two, and eggs start going bad around forty-two—well, you can do the math. A woman who delays childbearing also risks a decline in progesterone and estrogen, necessary hormones in childbearing. Without enough progesterone, the uterus cannot hold the fetus. Too, delays in childbearing allow for a longer time for the development of reproductive tract injury. In addition, ovaries can become more resistant to the stimulation needed to produce healthy eggs.

- **Polycystic ovary syndrome,** which affects about five million women.
- **Hormonal imbalances** could result in a lack of ovulation. Too much male hormone can be one of the problems. Dr. Schriock says at least 20 percent of women over forty fall into the hormonal imbalance category.
- **Too high or too low body fat.**
- **Chronic diseases, such as diabetes or hepatitis.**
- **Endometriosis.**
- **Medications.**
- **High rate of miscarriage.** Miscarriages are more

prevalent in older mothers than younger ones. (See the next chapter on pregnancy for an explanation.)

- **Impaired fecundity,** a related concern, is a medical term meaning the inability to carry a baby to full term.
- **Poor lifestyle factors,** i.e., the usual suspects: alcohol, cigarette smoking, illegal substance or prescription use.
- **Environmental factors** at the workplace or at home.
- **Sexually transmitted diseases** (STDs).
- **Fallopian tube blockage,** which accounts for about 20 percent of infertility.
- **Women who do not know what time of the month they are fertile.** Do you know how to tell if you are? Ask your gynecologist to explain.
- **Abnormal Pap smear.**
- **Ectopic pregnancies.**
- **Unknown or unusual causes.** This accounts for 20 percent and is a catchall category that includes uterine and cervical problems.

Diagnosing Your Problems

According to Schriock, a diagnosis of the cause of your infertility should be tailored to your age. "The workup is faster when the patient is older, since there is less time to play around," he says.

Your doctor should ask about your medical history: menstrual cycles (how long, how heavy, how far in between) and previous pregnancies, as well as infections or pain with intercourse and other related problems. A sperm test should be done on your partner. For any woman trying to get pregnant, a hormonal evaluation for progesterone and thyroid function should be taken followed by testing the quality of the patient's eggs, which is suggested for women over thirty. (The most common way to test egg quality is by measuring FSH and estradiol on day three of the menstrual cycle. This measures how hard the patient has to work to get her eggs to grow. To further assess egg quality, a patient can ask her doctor to perform the Clomid challenge test.) In addition, an ultrasound of the uterus and ovaries should be performed.

The general health of the patient should also be assessed via x-rays, EKG, blood tests, cardiac assessments, etc. The doctor should discuss the risks associated with later-in-life pregnancies (again, see the chapter on pregnancy) and your odds for developing those conditions.

It is also important to talk about expectations with the fertility specialist: expectations of success rate, cost, time frame and invasiveness, as well as an overview of the different ART procedures (see next page).

Next, psychological considerations, including the patient's motivation and the emotional impact of the procedures and risks of failure, should be laid on the table. If the fertility specialist you are seeing doesn't feel comfortable talking about the emotional impact of this event (or you don't feel comfortable talking with him or her), get a referral to a professional who specializes in this, i.e., an obstetrical psychotherapist.

Best of the Technologies Used Today

Dr. Rick Paulson, who helped the world's oldest known mother become pregnant, says we should not set up an arbitrary age limit as to who can and can't become pregnant. "Reproductive freedom is as basic as the freedom of speech," Paulson asserts. While there are no broad governmental guidelines as to the age limit, most fertility programs will not work with women older than fifty-one to fifty-five.

The fees for these procedures are high (you can spend twelve- to thirteen-thousand dollars plus medications on just one IVF cycle) and are infrequently paid for by health insurance, though the medications might be covered. Some states and some countries will pay for the procedure. Check with your local government to see if they do and what their guidelines are.

Treatments
Conventional IVF (In Vitro Fertilization)

While there is no guarantee that IVF will get you pregnant (the success rate drops by 50 percent each year after forty-two), it is the most successful of the infertility treatments available right now. This is especially true for the older mother.

IVF can be performed using a donor egg or using the patients own eggs. Both types of IVF function similarly. It involves fertilizing the egg(s) by the sperm outside of the mother's body in an artificial environment. First developed in 1977 in England, today tens of thousands of babies have been delivered as a result of IVF. IVF procedures used today are eons safer and simpler than when first developed.

The procedure is a big plus for older moms, because it increases the number of viable eggs. When a woman is in her twenties, she drops two hundred eggs each month; by the time she is forty, only five to ten eggs are produced monthly. Fertility drugs are used to stimulate the ovaries, thereby increasing the chances for a successful pregnancy. Next the eggs are retrieved from the ovary using ultrasound with sedation, but no general anesthesia. Fertilization of the eggs and culture of the embryos then takes place in the laboratory, followed by placement of the embryos into the uterus for implantation (known as "embryo transfer").

IVF can work if the infertility problem involves absent fallopian tubes or a tubal disease not treated otherwise; likewise endometriosis, male factor infertility when motility or count is low yet there are still enough active sperm, and unexplained infertility.

One cycle of IVF is usually a two-month process—that's two months from the time the decision is made to use IVF until the pregnancy test: one month to prepare, one month to try. Schriock warns that pregnancy rates over age forty run about 30 percent with subsequent delivery rates running only around 15 to 20 percent. "Therefore, 80 percent of the women who start this process are faced with the decision whether they want to do it again," he says. Your own fertility specialist should be able to tell you what he or she feels the chances are of a subsequent IVF procedure being successful.

According to *Fertility and Sterility Magazine,* taking oral contraceptives one month prior to IVF helps make the eggs more viable by giving the ovaries a rest in some cases. IVF specialists may also utilize birth control pills to facilitate the process.

IVF with Donor Eggs

While IVF is a miracle for many, the chances of pregnancy by IVF alone also diminishes with age, since it is the age and quality of the eggs that determines success. This is where the next step comes in: donor eggs.

"You can't fix an old egg, not even with IVF. The only way to replace it is with someone else's egg," Schriock informs. Donor eggs are retrieved from a donor with healthy, younger eggs. This is an older woman's best chance at pregnancy. Even women who are in menopause can get pregnant with this procedure. "Women who are menopausal," continues Schriock, "have a total ovarian failure which can have the highest success rate" because the problem is so identifiable so quickly: Infertility in menopause is caused by a lack of eggs.

Numerous donor eggs are retrieved at a time, so the patient can get several tries for the money. However, if there is a problem with the patient's uterus, carrying a baby will still not be possible. Contracting with a second woman to carry the baby can be an alternative. (See the chapter on surrogacy.)

The success rate of pregnancy enjoys an immediate boost when donor eggs are used: 40 to 60 percent become pregnant on the first try, about 76 percent after three tries.

IVF with a donor egg puts the patient in a unique position: She becomes the birth but not the genetic mother. As a result, this procedure can bring up difficult feelings. One woman we spoke with said she had a hard time bonding with a baby who did not have her genes.

However, when asked if they would rather be the birth or the genetic mother, women overwhelmingly said they would rather be the birth mother, according to the *Journal of Medical Ethics.*

"I chose egg donation over adoption or full-out surrogacy for a few reasons: The major one is I am the birth mother. Also, I can regulate how I care for myself while I am pregnant. I can't control that if another woman carried my baby." (*Note:* IVF with donor eggs can be considered a form of surrogacy, since the birth mother carries a fetus developed with her husband's sperm but with another woman's eggs. In "full-out" or traditional surrogacy, not only is another woman's eggs used, but the donor—or possibly a third woman—carries the baby to term.)

Another birth mother had a similar response: "What do you mean that baby is not 'mine'!" she gasps when asked. "I carried that baby and she came out of my body; how can she not be mine?"

Families formed by IVF and IVF with donor eggs are becoming commonplace: ads for donors abound in college newspapers and family publications all over. Check with your fertility specialist for the ways you can find a donor. Ask if the fertility specialist's program is open or closed, meaning will you have contact with the donor or not? Most programs let the recipient (that's you) decide.

Assisted Hatching

Assisted hatching is an IVF procedure wherein a hole is made in the outer coating of the embryo that has developed in the laboratory. This helps the embryo implant in the uterus (implantation also becomes more of a problem with the age of the mother). It is very noninvasive, so while the chances of it helping the embryo implant are not that enormous, it is worth the attempt.

Hormone/Fertility Medications

Some drugs commonly used are Clomid, Serophene and Gonal-F, Follistim and Repronex (some of these are given under the skin versus intramuscularly). They are used to stimulate egg production and are often used in conjunction with other therapies, especially IVF.

The next two procedures are not as commonly used as IVF and, rarely, if ever, used with donor eggs. Additionally, IVF is less invasive and has a better success rate.

Gamete Intra Fallopian Transfer (GIFT)

Gamete intra fallopian transfer is a variation on IVF, utilizing many of the same steps. The eggs and sperm are placed in the woman's fallopian tubes (via laparoscopy) to facilitate fertilization in the body. GIFT is available to women with normally functioning fallopian tubes and where male infertility is not the problem.

Zygote Intra Fallopian Transfer (ZIFT)

Zygote intra fallopian transfer is similar to GIFT, except fertilized *embryos* (called zygotes) are placed in healthy fallopian tubes. The eggs are retrieved in a similar manner as conventional IVF and cultured in the lab with sperm. The day after the retrieval, eggs that are determined to be fertilized but not yet dividing, are transferred to the fallopian tubes using laparoscopy under general anesthesia. ZIFT, as opposed to GIFT, provides your doctor direct information as to whether or not fertilization has been achieved.

Pre-Implantation Diagnosis

Once the embryo is formed, this test can confirm that only healthy embryos are transferred into the uterus, thereby eliminating the couple's fear of passing on genetic diseases (see Preconception chapter).

Embryo Freezing

A standard part of IVF treatment, during each retrieval more embryos than needed are collected; the extra embryos are frozen (embryo cyropreservation) and only the healthy ones are put back into the patient's uterus if an IVF cycle fails. When IVF is successful, the pregnant mother and her partner are then faced with what to do with the unimplanted embryos.

Thawing and unthawing frozen embryos for later use has been highly successful—not to be confused with freezing eggs, which is still very unsuccessful. Sometimes couples opt to thaw frozen embryos so they may have another child in later years; they can remain frozen for several years. Other couples volunteer the embryos to infertile couples.

The eventuality of what you will choose to do with the embryos not implanted should be planned for prior to undergoing the procedure.

Artificial Insemination

Once the backbone of the fertility industry, artificial insemination has lost its ground to the more high-tech (and more successful) procedures described in this chapter. There is only about a 10 to 15 percent chance of getting pregnant using artificial insemination; many reputable fertility specialists no longer offer this procedure. It's positive side is that it is much less costly than IVF.

Common Causes of Men's Infertility

Sperm abnormalities account for about 40 percent of infertility problems. Since male infertility problems are easier to treat, getting a workup for your partner should be the first step when a couple can't conceive. If the man's sperm count is low, that's almost a good thing.

No less than sixty-one surveys in the past years have shown that there is a rapid decrease in the number of sperm in men worldwide; the experts say this is caused in large part to environmental conditions such as pesticides and industrial chemicals. Male sperm count problems and blockages in the male reproductive system are commonly treated. Sometimes hormones or vitamin treatments (like zinc) are given to improve the quality and motility of sperm.

If your partner has had a vasectomy, reversal surgery is generally a simple and relatively commonplace procedure.

Below are more of the common causes of infertility in men.

- Sexually transmitted diseases (STDs) such as chlamydia
- Genital infection
- Mumps after puberty
- Hernia
- Undescended testicles
- Enlargement of the prostate
- Hormonal imbalance
- Varicose veins in genitals

A sperm specialist will take a history, conduct a physical including blood and sperm tests—from shape to motility (how well they move or "swim") to number and quality of motion, as well as hormone tests.

"For sure, there are much better odds if the couple's problem is the sperm. Even if there is one live sperm, we can inject it into the egg [see ICSI below]. Even men with *no* sperm can undergo a process to have the testicle biopsied with a very fine instrument to see if any pockets of sperm exist. If sperm exists, but it is not moving, we can test to see if it's still alive," Dr. Schriock says.

Treatment of Male Infertility
ICSI (Intracytoplasmic Sperm Injection)

This is a process that isolates a single sperm and injects it directly into the egg. The fertilized eggs are then transferred back into the uterus.

A relatively new technique, it was developed for couples with severe male factor infertility or couples who have failed to fertilize in a previously attempted IVF. It often allows couples with little hope to otherwise obtain fertilized embryos.

The woman undergoes ovarian stimulation (through medication) so that several mature eggs develop. The eggs are then aspirated (fluid removed) through ultrasound and incubated in the lab. The sperm sample is prepared by centrifuging (spinning sperm through a special medium for the purpose) which separates live sperm from sperm that is not usable. Very precise maneuvers are utilized to then pick up the single live sperm and inject it into the egg.

For couples with this infertility problem, there is a 70 to 80 percent success rate for *fertilization* which, of course, does not guarantee pregnancy—only the eggs determine that.

Schriock warns that ICSI may increase genetic problems. While it is a less than 1 percent concern (six out of one thousand babies versus two out of one thousand without it), your doctor should be queried on this.

Sperm "Banks"

Semen cryopreservation is the proper term. Sperm can be frozen from two sources: through ejaculates or through semen extracted in the operating room during a surgical procedure.

The sperm can be frozen for up to one year; if you are considering this procedure, you and your partner will need to discuss the frozen sperm's disposition after that point, just as you would talk about what to do with unused frozen embryos.

There seems to be no increase in birth defects from sperm that has gone through freezing and thawing versus freshly ejaculated sperm.

Emotional and Ethical Aspects

Grieving Process

A woman's decreasing chances of fertility—or the complete loss of it—is part of coming to terms with her own mortality. She needs to mourn the diminishing options to grow her family as she would any loss. "I was only forty-three, which seemed young to me; I couldn't believe it when the doctor told me I was infertile. I lapsed into a depression that took me a while to climb out of before I could think about what I wanted to do next," a new mother at last (via donor eggs) told me.

In order to move away from the grief, it is important to figure out what drives your desires to be a mother. What is your goal? Is it to become a parent even if the road to motherhood looks different from what you originally envisioned? Is it to become a parent strictly if you can give birth? Is it to have a baby with your DNA or no baby at all? It is important to talk these feelings through so you don't wind up resenting yourself or your partner. Look through the chapter on adoption for more information on grieving the loss of fertility.

The Monthly Ups and Downs

The nature of fertility treatments is a snaking of hope and disappointment. After being put through intensely invasive medical procedures month after month, you wait anxiously each cycle for the news you long for. Anger, sadness and resentment are common reactions when you don't get it. And if you finally do get your wish and become pregnant, well, even getting what you want can cause stress.

There is a good chance you will encounter some of these very natural feelings as you go through your own process in your quest for motherhood. Try to work with specialists who understand this, ones who will encourage you to examine your feelings. You want this time in your life to be filled with as much calm and happiness as possible.

Special Concerns of IVF with Donor Eggs or Sperm

In Dr. Schriock's experience, "Most women want to try other treatments before they opt for donor eggs. That's generally their last choice." This new technology is forcing us to find our way through a maze of new emotions and personal opinions. Among the things to consider: How will your relationship be affected if the sperm comes from your partner but the egg is not yours? Will you be able to bond with a baby who does not have your DNA? How will you tell your children about the circumstances of their birth—or your family and friends?

While the first two questions can only be answered by you, as for the latter, perhaps we can take a cue from the way adoption is handled by most adoptive families. Your child has every right to know the details of how he or she came into the world. Donor eggs, like adoption, are nothing to be ashamed of; conversely you and your family don't need to make it fodder for your breakfast table every day. Let your child know what you went through to get him or her because you wanted your child so much, then let the facts of his existence become part of the fabric of your lives, not the whole focus.

A good fertility specialist should talk to you about these concerns or recommend another professional for you to talk with.

At Last, Finding an Ethical Voice for Infertility Treatments

Where once any mention of getting babies by "fooling with mother nature" was greeted by upturned noses, today, having seen the happy results of ART for women and their families, people embrace it. A 2001 survey in *Family Circle Magazine* shows 67 percent of those surveyed said fertility treatments were a good thing, because they "helped people have babies." Only 18 percent believed they should be outlawed.

Other People's "Advice"

People can, without meaning to, belittle your plight and be unwittingly insensitive. Everyone who has ever given birth without the aid of ART (and even some who have) will tell you if only you would just relax, sleep on your left side, visualize yourself pregnant, etc., you will get pregnant. Try to keep their advice in perspective; it is rarely meant to be malicious. If you like, inform them that while you appreciate their advice, you need to proceed in the way that makes the most sense to you.

Treating Infertility Naturally

There are many herbalists, acupuncturists, practitioners of Chinese medicine, homeopathic doctors and others

involved in alternative medicine, each with di...
to aiding couples trying to conceive. The bare truth is that
if your infertility is the result of a "structural abnormality"
such as a blocked fallopian tube, nothing aside from surgery will fix it.

With that in mind, the following vitamins and herbs are
often considered for infertility problems:

- The B complex, especially B$_6$
- Selenium
- Vitamin C with bioflavonoids
- Vitamin A
- Calcium enriched with vitamin D
- Zinc (for male infertility as well)
- The antioxidants

Herbs thought to help include:

- Saw palmetto and true unicorn for your male partner
- Ginseng for both of you
- Black cohosh, chaste tree, cinnamon, dong quai,
  motherwort, squaw vine and wild yam root are also
  recommended for your infertility.

Choosing a Fertility Specialist

The fertility business is not regulated. It is a 2.6-billion-dollar business that seemingly mushroomed overnight. Where there were thirty clinics a decade and a half ago, there are upwards of three hundred in the United States now. As with anything else, it is not surprising there are allegations that some fertility clinics practice unsavory methods—methods that raise hopes falsely with their "frequent flier" money-back guarantees.

Don't Get Scammed

Respected experts warn to take the advertised success rates of a fertility doctor/clinic with a grain of salt. "There are many procedures still being used that are not effective," charges Schriock. These same clinics may advertise money-back guarantees and then require procedures not covered or not necessary. With the numbers of infertile women delaying childbearing until their later years, fertility clinics have come under criticism for competing for clients by sometimes exaggerating their success rates.

Here are some suggestions so you don't wind up an unwilling statistic:

- Hire a lawyer to review the contract.
- Ask yourself what your expectations are in terms of

success, cost, invasiveness and timeline. Then ask the clinic the same question.

- It has also been suggested that you should check the records of where your frozen embryos are stored to make sure they do not disappear.

What to Ask When Interviewing Fertility Specialists

- What is your success rate with women in my age group?
- What percentage of your practice is made up of women my age?
- How long will you work with me if I don't become pregnant in three months, six months, one year, etc.?
- Do you work with a psychotherapist who specializes in fertility issues or will you counsel me yourself about the emotional aspects?
- Will you help me look at egg donation versus adoption as an alternative?
- Can I develop ovarian cancer as a result of the treatments you advise for me?
- Please explain the fee schedule.
- Are there any rebates if the procedure does not work, and what procedures are specifically covered?
- Is the doctor board-certified?
- What is his or her training?

- How long has the program been around?
- How much say does the patient have in the treatment?
- Is it your sense that the clinic is open and patient with your questions?
- Can you tell me the pregnancy and miscarriage rates as well as the rates for birth defects?

In order to get an unbiased opinion, you might want to contact a nonprofit agency for a referral to a fertility specialist, like RESOLVE (you can find their contact info in the Resources chapter of this book).

The Newest Cutting-Edge Technologies

For years, the medical community would argue amongst themselves about how to convince women to not delay pregnancy. Apparently their pleas fell on deaf ears; women are having babies later and in larger numbers. So instead of making it the woman's problem, the fertility industry is racing the clock to meet the expectations of the older mother. With women delaying family life worldwide, reproductive technologists are in competition to find the ultimate answer to fertility problems. Here are some of their exciting developments:

1. **Diagnosing** to see if chromosomes are normal in an embryo rather than waiting for an amniocentesis.

2. **In vitro maturation:** Mature the eggs in vitro rather than taking shots and leaving eggs in the uterus and ovary.

3. **Freezing eggs:** This technology is close to being perfected. It means that women can freeze eggs when they are younger for later use.

4. **Lower miscarriage rates:** Three-quarters of embryos don't develop into babies. Now, thanks to London researchers, all twenty-three chromosomes can be tested. It is hoped that this procedure will lower the miscarriage rate and lead to increased birthrates.

6. Japan is working on an **artificial womb.**

7. Removing and **freezing ovaries** or ovary tissue. This procedure has been successful so far when reimplanted into monkeys.

8. A pill to **delay menopause:** Called a "researcher's dream" by its British developers, its purpose is to slow the number of eggs lost with each menstrual cycle.

CHAPTER 11

Pregnancy Beyond
Thirty-Five and After Forty

You've just put the phone down after the most amazing life-changing conversation you'll ever have. Your doctor called to say, "Get the baby's room ready. *You* are p-r-e-g-n-a-n-t!"

Translated this means: "Now the *real* work starts" (and that doesn't mean decorating). Being over thirty-five and into your forties is no longer an automatic barrier to a healthy pregnancy and a healthy bouncing baby, but it does require commitment on your part. With the right steps (which you must be taking if you are reading this book), there is every chance that you will have just as easy a time with your pregnancy as younger women— maybe even more so.

This chapter on pregnancy is offered as an educational *overview* without incorporating too much technical detail. Here are the considerations, conditions, tests and concerns for women over thirty-five and after forty—whether they are already pregnant, trying to become pregnant or trying to learn what a healthy pregnancy would mean for them. It is not meant to be a complete picture of your very personal condition. Your own doctor is the best source to get that.

If you've given birth before, your situation (meaning your body and how it reacts, as well as new tests available) is different from the last time you were pregnant, even if it wasn't that long ago: Here's where you can get current on recent findings.

If this is your first baby, terms used in this chapter may be somewhat familiar to you; but if you've only peeked over the shoulder of motherhood without diving in, your understanding may be minimal.

Good News!

Whether this is your first baby or not, over 90 percent of *all* births result in a healthy fetus. Later-in-life pregnancy is no longer routinely handed over to a perinatologist (an obstetrician specializing in high-risk pregnancies). When it comes to fulfilling the dream of a healthy, risk-free pregnancy, it's the general health of the mother, not age alone, that is the best indicator for success.

While the final advisor on the specific details of your unique situation, and that of your little bundle, will be your own doctor, barring unusual circumstances, your pregnancy can be a part of this 90 percent good news!

What's the Big Deal with Being Over Thirty-Five and Pregnant?

There is no magical, mystical thing that happens per se when a woman turns thirty-five to make her fall into the older pregnancy category. Then why is there a line drawn in the sand at thirty-five?

As best as can be deciphered, thirty-five got picked because it is the age that a woman's chances for having a baby with Down's syndrome is equal to having a miscarriage as a result of amniocentesis (about ½ percent). Because of this, the age of thirty-five became the watershed of "later" pregnancy; this despite the thousands of women thirty-five and forty-plus who have trouble-free pregnancies and healthy babies every year in ever-larger numbers.

A Return to Later Motherhood

As a matter of fact, pregnancy at thirty-five has become so commonplace that no one even bats an eye upon hearing of it anymore—in some circles, thirty-five is even considered young!

At the beginning of the last century, having babies past age thirty-five was more the norm than not. "The 1950s saw a decrease in the age of the mother, but before that women in their forties commonly gave birth; most likely, however, it was not her first child as it might be these days," explains sociologist Dr. Scott Coltrane of the University of California, Riverside.

Today, women who wait to have babies (or have babies again) are better educated than counterparts before; therefore, they take better care of themselves and their pregnancies. Ergo, they give birth to healthy, beautiful babies in ever-growing numbers. Typical age-related problems associated with pregnancies over thirty-five have been mostly dramatically diminished with the help of forethought and top-notch care.

A Little Bit About Childbirth Through the Ages

In the early ages, women gave birth by themselves. They wandered off to a secluded area of the tribe chosen by the soon-to-be-mother before she went into labor. This ritual progressed to childbirth assisted by other women in the tribe—usually female relatives who would accompany the pregnant woman to aid during delivery.

In the seventeenth and eighteenth centuries, these labor-coaching women became known as midwives.

Midwives were often thought to be witches by a suspicious male population left out of the mysterious birthing goings-on. That all changed in the 1820s when men entered the picture, literally, by presiding at deliveries. As a result, childbirth took on a new importance. Male physicians offered medical "advances" that included medications and forceps. Women were largely excluded from becoming physicians because they were believed to be un-educable about such matters; in addition, since the male doctors were in charge, female midwives were banned from the delivery rooms.

By 1910, obstetricians typically performed the births of the middle and upper classes; however, the majority of women were too poor to afford it and continued using midwives.

Much to everyone's surprise, a 1932 conference on childbirth found that European women who relied on midwives alone experienced a lower mortality rate for infants *and* mothers than American women who relied on physicians.

Today, women are choosing to combine a variety of delivery methods: While the use of midwives is again on the increase, so is the use of the newest technologies, like ultrasounds. The vast majority of babies are delivered in a hospital with a medical doctor performing the delivery and with Dad right at hand. And of course, women are now doctors in large numbers, though most midwives are also still female.*

Thanks to Dr. Coltrane for sharing this historical perspective.

Why Do Health Risks Increase with Age?

It's simply the fact of aging itself. No matter how great the care we give ourselves, the unequivocal truth is that we have more wear and tear on our bodies than women in their twenties, just because we've been here longer. This undeniable fact aside, much of what had been thought to be risks of later pregnancies is based on research that is old, reaching back to that period when the medical community referred to first-time mothers over thirty-five as "elderly primigravida."

Pregnancy health risks that exist for a woman thirty-five or older are comparable to the risks for teenage girls.

What the Experts Say About Later-in-Life Pregnancy

With so much advanced medical aid available to women who delayed having babies, the fear of first-time childbirth should be greatly decreased these days. (The fear of subsequent pregnancies should likewise be decreased, since they are in general easier than a first-time delivery, if all conditions are normal.)

While opinion can vary as to the care a later-in-life pregnant woman should receive, or even how the research should be interpreted, in the majority of cases, pre-pregnancy worries turn out to be too much ado about nothing. Most women who give birth over thirty-five and beyond forty have problem-free pregnancies and deliveries. "I was forty-three, and it was my first pregnancy. It was a piece of cake for me. I recovered a lot more quickly than women who were a lot younger than I was," one mom told us.

Dr. Hermina Salvador of Loma Linda University, and the obstetrician who delivered the child of the oldest known woman to give birth says, "Kudos to older moms. They are definitely making a choice. The quality of bonding between mother and child is excellent at this age. They have a different outlook. This child is very precious to them."

But why take chances with such an important and longed-for event, one you've most likely worked hard for? Get the best care you can afford and care for yourself in the best ways known to modern motherhood.

Ten Common Age-Related Pregnancy Concerns

(Note: The following special concerns are emphasized for pregnant women over thirty-five. This list is by no means meant to be a complete guide to your pregnancy. Please check with your doctor about concerns for pregnancy at any age.)

Many statistics that extrapolate conditions for women over thirty-five and forty do not take into account how much older mothers are willing to do to care for themselves when they are carrying a baby. So, while the odds of the concerns listed here can increase in direct correlation to the age of the mother, it does not mean that you will encounter any of these just because of your age.

1. **Miscarriage:** At least 20 percent of *all* pregnancies result in miscarriage (or spontaneous abortion). Some experts even surmise that nearly half of all pregnancies result in miscarriage but go unnoticed since they happen so early—in the embryonic stage or even earlier as the zygote (defined as the cell produced by the two gametes—basically, the sperm and the egg), before the cells divide. Still others believe that the numbers of miscarriages don't increase; it's just that our methods of being able to spot miscarriages earlier on have improved.

   Miscarriage can result in a devastating emotional aftermath, especially for women who have waited to get pregnant. "I miscarried just after a few weeks. I was forty-two at the time. After the miscarriage, I was distraught. I had gotten in touch with how much I really wanted a child, and I couldn't let go of it," a forty-four-year-old newly pregnant (again) future mom reports.

   Many doctors have concluded that miscarriage occurs as nature's way of aborting a fetus that carries a life-threatening problem or one that would impede normal growth and development.

   Miscarriage rates for women over thirty-five are

higher (18 percent between thirty-five and thirty-nine) than for younger women, especially in the first trimester where most miscarriages take place. In fact, 53 percent of miscarriages happen in women over forty.

2. **Pre-eclampsia (also known as toxemia):** Diagnosed as a sudden increase in weight caused by water retention, pain under the right rib cage, headaches, high blood pressure or protein in the urine, pre-eclampsia is about 1.5 times more prevalent in women over thirty-five, teenage girls and women bearing their first child. Toxemia generally occurs during the last trimester of pregnancy; it's easy to spot a pregnant woman with toxemia, because she has a puffy look and swollen hands and feet.

   In a nutshell, toxemia means that less nourishment is getting to the fetus. While the exact cause of this condition is under deliberation, it is evident that women who smoke, eat poorly and don't stick to their ob/gyn appointments—in general, women who don't take care of themselves—have the highest incidence of toxemia. In general, toxemia can be handled without disrupting the health of the mother or child. Check with your doctor to see where she stands on the controversy about taking baby aspirin, if you appear to be at risk for toxemia. If you develop this condition, your doctor may advise bed rest.

A case of very severe toxemia can mean hospitalization to guard your health.

Eat well. The little life you are carrying depends on you.

3. **Placenta Previa:** This is a condition where the placenta is low in the uterus and covers the internal opening of the cervix either in part or in its entirety. It is more common in smokers as well as older women: Women over thirty-five have twice the chance of developing this condition. The odds increase the older the mother. Chances also increase with twins. However, this condition occurs in only about 10 percent of first time pregnancies; if this is your fifth full-term birth, your chances are one in twenty.

   Bleeding without pain is the main symptom. Ask your doctor to assess your risk; once pregnant, an ultrasound can confirm if you have the condition. Your treatment will depend on how far along you are and how much bleeding there is.

   There is a possible risk to the fetus as well.

4. **Stroke/Hypertension:** In simple terms, hypertension is raised blood pressure. Hypertension is on the shortlist of common problems (along with diabetes and anemia) for all women, regardless of age at pregnancy. However, there does appear to be a higher incidence in older women.

5. **Gestational Diabetes:** You will also hear this condition referred to as gestational glucose intolerance and maternal diabetes. Diabetes is one of the top-three problems that crop up in pregnancies, regardless of the age of the mother. Being overweight can cause the onset of gestational diabetes. Have you gained weight recently (which is not uncommon as we age and gets harder to take off)? The concern is that with diabetes, placental problems can increase and result in premature babies. With treatment and early diagnosis, the condition is usually not a threat to either baby or mother.

6. **Cesarean:** Mention C-sections and watch women's faces cringe. Mortality rates for women are higher with C-sections than with vaginal delivery, though still small. C-sections are also more painful than vaginal deliveries, require longer hospital stays and have a higher risk of post-delivery infection. Controversial for women of any age, it is by far the most controversial procedure in connection with older mothers and their pregnancies. Cesareans occur about twice as frequently in women in the over-thirty-five age group than in the traditional childbirth years of twenty to twenty-nine. The exact reason for this is hard to pin down, though one often stated is that C-sections require a shorter time than vaginal deliveries and, rightly or wrongly, can be scheduled anytime, thereby

freeing up the busy doctor to attend to other business.

It can be difficult to clarify if C-sections are performed for the doctor's peace of mind or because they are truly needed; only your doctor knows for sure. Research is highly contradictory, and doctors say they prefer C-sections when there is a risky delivery or an older mother is having a first-time baby. What *is* known is that C-sections are on the rise: 22 percent of *all* deliveries are now C-sections.

What is a cesarean? A cesarean is when the baby is removed from the mother's abdomen versus vaginally, the latter being the natural way. Called everything from a medical fad to a blessing for high-risk pregnancies, the good news is that women who have had a C-section no longer are required to have one in all subsequent births.

As a backlash to the high incidence of cesareans in recent years, some doctors and hospitals are going back to more natural methods. For instance, one Chicago hospital's nursing staff helps the mother walk more frequently while in labor to encourage natural descent of the fetus; nurses are also expected to be more hands-on especially for first-time moms, of which many are in the over-thirty-five category.

Some women report that cesareans are sprung on them as they are wheeled into the delivery room. To avoid an unwanted surprise, make sure you discuss C-sections thoroughly with your obstetrician prior to your delivery date.

7. **Multiple Births:** Since the onset of the widespread usage of fertility drugs, multiple births have increased for older women. While the chances of any woman giving birth to twins are one in eighty-nine without fertility drugs, it doubles after fertility drug use (one in forty-three). The rate for triplets has increased from one in six-thousand to one in four-teen-hundred pregnancies.

   But even without drugs, there is an increase in odds that you will have multiple babies the older you are: A fifty-four-year-old grandmother of eight gave birth to triplets in early 2000 without any drugs; actress Adrienne Barbeau had twins at fifty-one, also without the aid of fertility drugs.

   If you are expecting to be doubly, triply—or more—blessed, you might be automatically relegated to the high-risk pregnancy category. Multiple births often bring a higher incidence of premature babies and the concerns that ensue as a result (such as cerebral palsy).

   Since low birthweight is also often associated with premature babies, multiples may, too, be the reason why there is a reported slight increase in the number of low-weight babies born to older mothers.

8. **Longer Recovery Time:** The older you are, the longer it takes to bounce back to your pre-pregnancy shape, even if your pre-pregnancy shape was pretty terrific.

You may be more tired and have a slower metabolism. Sleep deprivation takes a harder toll on older than younger mothers.

Exercising before, during and after pregnancy (with your doctor's consent), as well as eating right (see below), are some of your best aids in getting back to shape as soon as possible.

9. **Body Changes:** A host of changes occur as a result of pregnancy, from tiny amounts of calcium being leached from your bones to the more visible, like a thicker waistline (breastfeeding can help) and saggier breasts. Women who give birth put on an average six pounds more than women who don't over a five-year period. A typical pregnancy weight gain is thirty pounds: 7.5 pounds of that are the baby (though older mothers have larger babies, 9 pounds and over), another 10 pounds are increased fluids (like blood and amniotic) and 5.5 pounds comes from the uterus, breasts and placenta. This leaves 7 pounds, including the maternal store of fat, protein and nutrients for the baby.

Since it is harder to take weight off the older we get, and since osteoporosis is a big concern starting around the time of menopause, a woman who gets pregnant in her middle years needs to be aware of these potential side effects. But give yourself a break.

Don't expect to lose weight overnight nor tighten every muscle back to its pre-pregnancy tautness. You just had a baby—and at your age!

On the bright side, if your period was irregular prior to pregnancy, it will probably become regular afterward. Also, your chances for ovarian and breast cancer are lowered.

10. **Left-handed babies:** Women over forty have a higher birth rate of babies who are left-handed. Some research connects left-handedness with an increase in birth stress, prolonged labor, difficulty in breathing at birth, low birth weight or the trauma of being a twin or triplet. Since multiples are more likely in later-in-life moms, this alone may account for more left-handed babies.

Left-handed babies are also an inch shorter in general and three pounds lighter than babies who favor their right hands. None of these things is considered any sort of problem; as a matter of fact, in some circles, left-handedness is considered to be the mark of creativity and genius.

Pregnant Again After Many Years

"No matter what you hear, the second pregnancy is harder especially if it comes years after the others," says one forty-five-year-old pregnant-again mother of a twelve-year-old son. Since your muscles are already stretched, you will most likely start showing sooner. You might suffer an increase in backaches: The ligaments that hold the uterus are now spread out. There is more of a chance that you will carry the baby lower which means more back pain. Feeling more tired than you remember the first time could be in part because you have the other child(ren) to care for, in addition to being pregnant.

What's the up side? You are probably not as worried about every twist, turn and pain, since you've done this before. Labor is generally shorter than the first time (cut in about half). And who knows better than you what a miracle you are about to experience?

Genetic Counseling

Are you concerned about passing on a disease or disorder that runs in your family? Do either you or the child's father belong to an ethnic group that commonly contracts a high-risk disorder, such as Tay-Sachs or sickle-cell anemia? Are you a close *blood* relation to your partner (e.g., a cousin)?

Ideally, genetic testing should be ordered in the pre-conception stage (see The Preconception Checkup chapter); however, if you are worried about any of these risks and are already pregnant, it is not too late to order tests specific to each concern.

Special Tests to Consider

Head off the anxiety you feel about pregnancy tests by educating yourself about them. Always ask when the results will be in the doctor's hands, how you will be notified, who you can talk to if you haven't heard anything as of the appointed time and what the outcomes will mean to you.

Keep your partner informed as to the tests you'll need, what the possible outcomes are and what, if anything, can be done about less-than-perfect results.

Down's Syndrome

Down's syndrome is the only birth defect that can be directly correlated to the age of the mother and coincidentally the age of her eggs. New research also indicates that the age of the father (especially if he's in his fifties or older) can also contribute to the incidence of Down's syndrome (because of longer exposure to environmental factors, etc.).

Down's syndrome occurs when there is an extra chromosome causing a variety of physical and mental retardation effects, which generally include facial features that denote Down's syndrome.

When a woman gives birth at age thirty, the chances of her baby developing Down's syndrome is 1 in 885; at thirty-five, 1 in 378; at forty, 1 in 109; at forty-five, 1 in 32. While this sounds high statistically, it translates to only a 1 percent chance that a baby born to a forty-year-old mother will have Down's syndrome. Therefore, even at these odds in your mid-forties, your chances of giving birth to a baby *without* Down's syndrome are almost perfect—96 to 98 percent. If you are concerned about Down's syndrome, talk to your doctor about undergoing an amniocentesis or CVS test (see below). Also, talk to your partner to decide what course you will take if your baby does have Down's syndrome.

Answering this question might help you determine if you should have an amniocentesis or not.

If Down's syndrome is a concern, talk about the following four tests with your doctor. Ask which he or she believes is more reliable and which he or she believes is safer. Always inquire as to how many amnios the medical professional who will be performing yours has done. The more, the merrier, for your peace of mind.

1. **Amniocentesis:** Amniocentesis became available in 1968 and has grown in use since then. This test can only be performed once you are pregnant. It is the definitive test to tell if your fetus is carrying Down's syndrome.

   Amnios are usually performed about sixteen to eighteen weeks into fetal development; results can take ten days to three weeks. A needle is placed through the mother's abdomen and into the uterine cavity, where a small amount of amniotic fluid in which the fetus is floating is withdrawn for analyzing. Whatever cells are gathered are then grown under lab conditions and their chromosomal makeup is microscopically photographed and examined. A normal female fetus will be 46XX; normal male is 46XY. When there is an extra chromosome, one missing or something else in its place, trisomy 21 or Down's syndrome is the likely result.

The risk of losing a fetus via miscarriage as a direct result of the amniocentesis test is about 1 per every 250 procedures.

About 95 percent of the women who undergo amniocentesis get the reassuring news that their baby is developing without chromosomal abnormalities.

2. **CVS: Chorionic Villus Sampling** is usually performed between nine-and-a-half to eleven weeks in the first trimester and therefore earlier than amnio. It should be used in conjunction with ultrasound for safety (as with the other tests listed here). Its purpose is not limited to determining chromosomal abnormalities but also for determining the sex of the baby. There are two ways to perform this procedure: one is with a needle through the abdomen, the other with a catheter in the cervix. A sample of tissue is then analyzed. Results can take as long as an amnio. Risks include a higher incidence of miscarriage as well as the possibility of causing damage to the limbs of the fetus.

3. **AFP:** By 1983, AFP testing (Alphafetoprotein is produced in the fetus' liver and is also present in the
   mother's blood) was being widely performed. It is a
   blood test performed between the fifteenth and twentieth weeks. A very low amount of AFP may mean your
   baby is afflicted with Down's syndrome. A high reading
   could mean spina bifida or other conditions (none of
   which have been proven to have a higher incidence in
   women over thirty-five). Not as reliable a test as CVS or
   amniocentesis, only 20 percent of Down's syndrome
   babies are detected via AFP. However, an amnio can be
   used in conjunction with AFP, if called for.

   Triple AFP Screen: A newer and extended version
   of AFP, this test screens estrogen, HCG (pregnancy
   hormones), as well as AFP. It is claimed that 60
   percent of Down's syndrome fetuses can now be
   recognized through this test.

4. **Fetal Nuchal Translucency Screening:** This test was
   developed at the University of California, San
   Francisco, to allow doctors to detect chromosomal
   abnormalities much earlier. It measures the fluid accu-
   mulated in the neck that, if abnormal swelling or
   enlargement occurs, indicates a defect. This procedure
   is performed during the first trimester (ten to fourteen
   weeks) and predicts with 80 percent accuracy Down's
   syndrome. It can also alert doctors and mothers to

increased risk of other worrisome conditions, such as heart defects.

Ultrasound

Ultrasound diagnosis has become the standard for *all* prenatal checkups today, regardless of the age of the mother; for older mothers, it can be a reassuring godsend. Ultrasound can alert a physician to problems that may require an amniocentesis for chromosomal problems, in addition to a whole host of other possible concerns, including heart, facial or skeletal defects, as well as neural tube defects. Ultrasound can also tell your doctor how the baby is growing. Ultrasound is also used in conjunction with amniocentesis or CVS to help make those procedures safer. It is generally without risk to the mother or the fetus.

A High APGAR Score Will Not Help Your Baby Get into the University of Your Choice

Then why does everyone brag about it? APGAR (named for a female anesthesiologist who developed it in 1952) is a benchmark used all over the world. It evaluates five vital signs—muscle tone, respiratory effort, crying, color and pulse (which indicate how well the circulatory system is doing) and reflex irritability (showing the baby's response to external stimulation). These five markers tell the doctor how the baby is doing *within the first few moments of life*—period. Each category is assigned a number from 0 to 2. The results of the scoring add up to a maximum of ten. A low score after one minute of birth is generally not something to get overly concerned about; the baby is usually retested after some slight intervention. The new score most likely will be seven or higher.

If your baby is high risk, he or she will probably be given an additional test, the Neonatal Behavioral Assessment Scale, at a later date.

Increasing Your Odds for a Healthy Outcome

Prenatal diagnosis started in the 1950s and has boomed into a regular course of business for every thinking pregnant woman regardless of age. Ever-expanding technology is available to evaluate the unborn fetus—and risks to mothers—from virtually every angle.

One of the best ways to increase your odds for a healthy outcome is an old-fashioned remedy: Get a doctor you trust. Will your doctor be there with you throughout, answering questions and monitoring your progress, proceeding cautiously but not reacting automatically about any conditions that arise? Can you talk easily with him or her, or are you made to feel foolish when you ask questions or express concerns?

When you choose an obstetrician, you are hiring someone to perform a very precious task—helping you become a mother. Interview the doctor, and check references so you can feel confident in your doctor's ability. This is the very least you would do when choosing a car mechanic or veterinarian, isn't it?

Questions to Ask and Observations to Make About Your Obstetrician

- Where does the doctor perform his or her deliveries? Call to see if you can go to the hospital to check it out. Ask the staff if they would use Dr. So-and-So personally? Ask the doctor for patient references in your age group.
- Will this doctor perform your preconception exam?

Will he or she include special tests because of your age?

- What percentage of patients does this doctor have in the over thirty-five and forty age range?

- How often will the doctor see you during your pregnancy? Is this more frequently than a younger woman would be seen?

- What is his or her opinion of amniocentesis? Will this doctor insist you have one? If you decide to end the pregnancy as a result of your amnio, will your doctor have any objections on a personal level?

- What about cesareans? Will you automatically be given one because of age? In the event your own doctor cannot perform your delivery, how does the hospital where you will be delivering the baby feel about C-sections?

- How long will you have to wait for return phone calls if you have questions in between appointments?

- Under what circumstances would the doctor feel it necessary to induce labor? (FYI: According to the National Center for Health Statistics, the number of births by induced labor is on the rise, jumping from 9 percent in 1989 to double that by the end of the 1990s.) Labor should never be induced for the sake of "convenience," but only in cases where continuing the pregnancy is a risk to the mother or fetus.

- Will you automatically be considered high risk if you

are carrying multiple fetuses? Will you automatically have a C-section?

- Get a sense of how your obstetrician is reacting to your questions. Is he or she open-minded and encouraging, making sure you get all your concerns addressed, or does the doctor possess a "me doctor, you patient" attitude? If the latter is true, it may be time for you to find another obstetrician.

Caring for Yourself While Pregnant

There is a new life forming, one who is depending on the wise choices you will be making for both of you from now on: watching what you eat, what you do and even what you think.

The Big Three No-No's That You Already Know-Know

- **Alcohol:** Fetal alcohol syndrome, which is the cause of a variety of physical and mental distresses, is easily avoided just by not drinking alcohol while trying to get pregnant, during your pregnancy or while you are nursing.
- **Smoking:** Smoking cigarettes or cigars—or even being around anyone who does—is something you will want to give up permanently. Once your baby is born, a

smoke-free environment gives him or her a better shot at having healthy lungs.

• Drugs of any kind (see the following page).

It's Important to Agree with and Follow Your Doctor's Advice

This includes not taking any over-the-counter *or* prescription drugs (including accutane acne medicine), unless the doctor prescribing it knows you are pregnant and is aware of any special circumstances.

Since you have carefully chosen a doctor you feel comfortable with, this will not be a problem, because he or she will have your full confidence and cooperation, right?

Well, with one proviso.

It's Your Pregnancy

You are the one it's all happening to, so if a test is ordered or a suggestion is made that you do not understand or are not comfortable with, take the time to talk to your doctor about why he or she feels it's important for you. If you still decide against it, you must inform your doctor, so he or she can take the proper next steps. Remember, your bottom line is a safe pregnancy and healthy baby.

Caring for Yourself Naturally

1. **Diet and Nutrition:** Research at last bears out what many healthy eaters have known for years: What you ingest prior to, as well as during your pregnancy, and of course while you are nursing, affects not only your health but the health of your baby.

   One way you can eat well includes adding more fish to your diet. Fish will aid in the baby's brain development: salmon and tuna are perfect sources. Fish is loaded with omega-3 fatty acids.

   However, this is a double-edged sword. Some fish (king mackerel, shark, swordfish and tuna in large quantities, for example) is thought to be a risk for mercury contamination.

   An alternative healthy fat to eat is olive oil.

   Eating dark green leafy vegetables like spinach or dark green lettuces adds a variety of vitamins and minerals safely to your diet. Likewise, citrus fruits such as oranges, grapefruits and lemons (lemon juice in water will help keep nausea under control); they are loaded with vitamin C, while melons like cantaloupe are known for their vitamin A content. Nuts of all kinds, as well as seeds such as sunflower, whole beans and tofu are an excellent source of protein.

   A Word About Herbs:

   Herbs can be a wonderful resource for women under any condition, especially with the symptoms of pregnancy. Be sure to advise your doctor if you are going to use herbs (or vitamins not prescribed). This is the only way your doctor can keep a complete picture of your health.

Folic Acid and Vitamin Supplements:

Many of you are probably already taking vitamins every day; if not, you will be given a prescription for prenatal vitamins once you become pregnant.

A study in the late 1990s showed that six out of nine prenatal vitamins did not meet the dissolution standards set by the U.S. Pharmacopoeia (that's what the USP printed on vitamin labels stands for). The standards require that 75 percent of the folic acid in a pill be released within an hour after taking it. The USP recommends: 1) Choose a single-ingredient folic acid vitamin that contains a minimum .4 milligrams. 2) Take the vitamin on a full stomach; and 3) Make sure the label states that your particular tablet helps protect against neural defects.

Taking folic acid when pregnant is said to cut spinal and brain defects by almost half. Found naturally in citrus fruits, beans, tuna, eggs and leafy green vege-tables, many grain products (like whole grain breads) also now include folic acid.

Many excellent books have been written about nutri-tion and pregnancy. One of my favorites is *What to Eat*

When You Are Expecting by Arlene Eisenberg et al. As a matter of fact, the entire *What to Expect* series is excellent.

2. **Special Treats:** Carrying your baby for nine months is hard work. It's time to treat yourself.

   - Nothing says lovin' like a good massage; who kneads those knots?

   - If you are feeling discomfort, get out of the house and try walking it off in the fresh air.

   - Exercise and deep breathing will keep you practically stress-free. And it feels terrific! Don't forget your Kegel exercises as well, to keep your vaginal muscles in good shape.

   - Prenatal exercise classes feel especially great. "I took one in a swimming pool and it was wonderful," one mom over thirty-five says of her second pregnancy.

   - This is also a great time to develop or expand your spiritual life (see the chapter "In It for the Long Haul"). Whatever your personal beliefs or philosophy, practicing them now will not only help you through the rough spots while you are pregnant, but will solidify a family foundation once your child arrives.

   - Another special treat to consider is hiring a doula, a trained labor coach who supports you during the birth as well as after the baby comes home. One study found that women who used doulas were less likely to need an epidural. Doulas do not replace midwives or doctors (or dads!).

Pregnancy and Your Emotions

Having a baby is a very big life change, especially when you have waited, have tried getting pregnant for a while or are restarting childrearing after a period of time. The news that you are really, *actually* pregnant can come as a shock and a blessing rolled into one. As your fear and excitement battle it out, your emotions leave you overwhelmed.

The push and pull you feel is not relegated only to the moment you find out you are pregnant; there are plenty of other passing thoughts to drive you nuts throughout the nine months: "Will my baby be all right?" "What was I thinking to do this?" "Will I be too old to have another one?" Hormones play with your emotional equilibrium throughout your pregnancy. They play not only on your body, but your mind. High estrogen and progesterone levels affect your nervous system.

If your worse thoughts start getting the better of you, turn to help. For instance, waiting for the results of an amniocentesis can add stress to your stress. To help deflate the fears, gather a network of women who are in the same boat at the same time (or have been there before) that you can check in with when the emotional going gets rough—when your mind might start playing tricks on you. "It really helped to have a friend who had gone through it last year. She knew to call me every day, and every day we had the same conversation. 'Just keep reminding yourself that most amnios turn out okay,' she told me. I got through and she was right! My baby was perfectly healthy," says a more relaxed forty-seven-year-old mother of a two-year-old healthy boy.

It's not unusual to freak yourself out and have a good old-fashioned crying jag for no other reason except for your ever-expanding tummy. Focus on thoughts that lift your spirits, like all the things that are in your favor.

Pregnancy can also make you feel good: Hormones can be responsible for feelings of elation and joy—as well as jolts of brilliance. A University of Richmond study shows that pregnancy hormones can actually help a woman learn and remember things.

Attend childbirth classes and encourage your partner to come as well. Everyone benefits, especially you and the baby. Aside from what you'll learn, it's a great place to share your fears as well as be comforted, relax and get geared up for the new life growing in you.

If you feel too down too often (the times when a cup of tea or dumping on a girlfriend doesn't ease the blues), consider talking to a professional who can help you get a perspective. Ask your obstetrician to recommend someone who works with pregnant women.

Working While Pregnant

Not that long ago, pregnant women were considered a blight on the workplace. Tummies growing with new life were to be hidden at home.

Today, if a woman thinks of working while she is pregnant, it is her health and pocketbook that are the determining factors. Certainly dressing for the occasion is no longer a problem—whole businesses have thrived dressing today's pregnant woman smartly.

What will you do about working while pregnant? Will you cut back on hours, work for just a few months or not at all? These are questions only you, your doctor, your partner and your bank account can answer.

Remember, you are not superwoman.

Expect Positive Outcomes

Every doctor I spoke with and every piece of research I came across all concluded the same thing: If you are in good shape to begin with, eat well, exercise and have gone for a preconception checkup, your chances of delivering a healthy baby are as good over thirty-five and forty as they are at any age.

CHAPTER 12

Choosing Motherhood Through Surrogacy

Like many of the now widely accepted alternatives to remedy childlessness, surrogacy remains little understood. "The public's perception of surrogacy is the opposite of what it's really like, as those who have done it know," says Kay Johnson, forty-seven, and the mother of two children through surrogacy. She is also the president of the Organization of Parents Through Surrogacy. But despite the public's misconception, the use of surrogacy has shown a healthy growth in popularity: About ten thousand babies have arrived in the last twenty-five years to help form new families, thanks to surrogacy.

Surrogacy allows the contracting couple

(you) to be very involved in their child's birth. Its success relies on combining several techniques which allow the surrogate mother to carry the baby for the contracting (a.k.a. as "intended") couple. Adoption by the intended mother follows the birth of the child.

How Surrogacy Works
It Started with a Desire to Help . . .

In 1976, lawyer Noel Keane (referred to as the "father" of surrogacy) had a simple idea: Some women can get pregnant, some who want to cannot; why not have them help each other? With this thought, a whole new door opened for women.

Surrogacy marries the concerns of infertility with the concept of adoption. In its basic form, a woman who is infertile (along with her partner, if there is one) contracts with another woman, who becomes known as the surrogate. The surrogate becomes impregnated medically by the infertile couple's sperm, thereby allowing the child to be biologically related to at least one parent. Upon delivery of the baby, the gestational or biological mother relinquishes her parental rights and gives the baby up to the biological father and his wife, who are the contracting/intended couple.

If you choose surrogacy, you are in good company: Many women have done so before you. Most recently, actress/model Cheryl Tiegs became a mother again at fifty-three via twin boys delivered by a surrogate. Already a mother to an eight-year-old son, she tried to conceive for a year. Her husband's sperm and her own eggs were used. Soap opera actress Diedre Hall (*Days of Our Lives*) was forty-two the first time she become a mother through surrogacy. She became an immediate advocate, repeating the process to become a mother a second time.

Public Controversy

In 1986, surrogate Mary Beth Whitehead (of the infamous "Baby M" case) put surrogacy on the map but under a very negative light: Whitehead changed her mind about giving up rights to the baby she bore for the couple she was under contract with.

The courts eventually ordered the biological/contracting father and his wife full custody. But the face of surrogacy changed in the public's perception; some media even charged it was akin to "baby selling."

Fortunately, today's view of surrogacy has shifted. A *Family Circle* (September 2000) survey showed 68 percent of the survey participants believe that a surrogate should not be able to keep the child if she changes her mind.

Types of Surrogacy

There can be as many as five people involved in a surrogacy birth: the egg donor, the contracting mother and father, the gestational mother (who can be a different woman from the egg donor) and sperm donor, if not the contracting father. Here are the most common forms of surrogacy:

1. **Traditional Surrogacy** involves artificially inseminating the gestational (birth) mother with the contracting father's sperm.

2. **Gestational Surrogacy** is when the egg of the contracting mother (you) and the sperm of the contracting father are used to create an embryo that is implanted into the gestational surrogate, because it is deemed the contracting mother will not be able to carry the baby to term. With this method, the child has the contracting mother's and father's (or sperm donor's) DNA.

3. **Gestational Surrogacy and Egg Donation:** The gestational mother carries the embryo developed with a donor egg and sperm from the contracting father.

Less frequently, a sperm donor can also used with any of these methods.

Getting Started

Since there are no across-the-board governmental restrictions in regard to surrogacy, do your homework before signing on the dotted line. If you are using a surrogacy agency instead of an independent arrangement, pick the agency that most closely matches your personal needs. Check into the agency's policies on age or marital restrictions, as well as fees charged. Determine if the surrogacies they work with are open or closed.

"Always use the best professionals you can find to make sure every detail is done right. It's not going to save you money to do otherwise, since you will wind up paying thousands later to fix what should have been done right in the first place," Johnson advises.

Here are other things to consider:

Agencies

One of the benefits of going through an agency is it generally has a wide pool of surrogates to choose from. Check into how surrogate candidates are screened: You want them to be screened medically as well as psychologically. Make sure that surrogates are not on welfare and therefore in it strictly for the money. How are surrogates paid? One lump sum? Monthly? (FYI: Surrogates should never be given any information about *your* finances.) Does she have medical insurance? Are there support groups for the surrogates used by the agency? Will you be privy to your surrogate's medical records?

Many surrogacy agencies can also connect you with an egg donor for purposes of IVF (see the chapter on fertility for more about IVF with egg donation), if you want to carry the baby yourself.

Privately Arranged

Many women have used someone they know as their surrogate—close friend, cousin, sister, even a mother-in-law! If you are going this route, hire a lawyer who works with surrogates regardless (or perhaps especially) if you are using a relative or friend.

Legal Issues

Before any medical procedures are started, there must be something "in writing" for the protection of everyone (don't forget we are talking about creating a human life). The contract should spell out the rights, responsibilities and intentions of all concerned. It is imperative that certain issues are covered in the contract: Most important is the finalizing of the parental rights of the surrogate after the child is born. If the surrogate has a husband, ask your lawyer if he should likewise be mentioned in the contract.

While putting everything in writing can go a long way to minimize stress during this emotional time, not every governmental body recognizes contracts between surrogates and contracting parents. Check with yours (state, country) to see if an agreement is enforceable. While some states in the United States make surrogacy agreements illegal, it thrives in Britain and many other European countries.

Fees

Mary Beth Whitehead was paid ten thousand dollars in 1986; today, surrogacy costs can top over fifty thousand dollars, but it is generally closer to thirty-thousand dollars, which includes all fees.

Emotional Issues

The agency you choose should offer counseling by a professional psychotherapist to both the surrogate and you. You are going through an experience that not only have *you* not gone through before, but in all likelihood, most of the people you know have not either. Therapy prepares you for the process. It is crucial.

Postpartum counseling is also a consideration until the need dwindles.

Your Fears

Will the surrogate change her mind? Will I be able to bond with a child who is not mine or who I didn't give birth to? How will everyone I know feel about the baby? These thoughts are normal for anyone undergoing an experience like becoming a mother through surrogacy; mothers who adopt or go through IVF can also have similar crazy-making thoughts. The bottom line is you can't allow yourself to over-shadow the impending joy with impending fears. "I did a lot of soul-searching," one forty-seven-year-old mother through surrogacy concludes. "And the decision is right for us."

If surrogacy is right for you, you will know it.

Meeting and Matching with a Surrogate

How do you pick a surrogate? "It's a gut feeling," says one mom. "I wasn't looking for someone who looked like me. I knew enough to know there were more important values," opined another. What qualities do you want your surrogate to have? How would you describe yourself to a potential surrogate? How much contact do you want with the surrogate? Is your surrogate married? Does she have children already, and if so, how will she tell her children about her experience with you? Is her family supportive?

Do you want an open or closed program? Relationships with the surrogate vary and details of during-the-pregnancy and after-the-birth-contacts need to be worked out between all parties *in advance*. Most contracting mothers want to go to every doctor's appointment and be at the birth. Typically the surrogate and contracting mother will keep in touch with each other by phone.

Some issues that need to be discussed: Will you require the surrogate to undergo an amniocentesis? What will you and your partner do if the fetus has Down's syndrome or another genetic disorder?

Why Do Surrogates Do It?

Many surrogates already have their own children and have a higher calling to share their fortune. "I was lucky that I could get pregnant. I have three beautiful kids, and I wanted to share that with someone who wasn't able to have any," says one surrogate.

"I can't imagine someone not being able to have kids if they want one," another surrogate offers.

Telling Your Child, Telling Others

One mother through surrogacy (with children ages six and three) tells her children that all babies come from an egg and sperm. In letting them know this, they understand that they are the same as everyone else. As time goes on, more details can be revealed. As in adoption, saying, "Mommy couldn't carry you, so your birth mother did" sums it up in an easy-to-understand and truthful package for younger ones.

As for telling others outside of your family, how much information they are told is a personal choice. You may not know how you feel about sharing the news until your baby was born. Many couples who have become parents through surrogacy report feeling "surprised" that they wanted to let the world know, once they became parents.

Family Values

With little pun intended, surrogacy is still in its infancy, along with many new assisted reproduction technologies (ARTs). As with most new ideas in history, controversy comes with the territory—at least until it is understood better. The whole field of ARTs exists because women past thirty-five have a strong desire for family life.

What better family values could you ask for?

CHAPTER 13

Forming Your Family Through Adoption

Not every woman gets pregnant; this is especially true of women in midlife. For those would-be mothers (or those would-be mothers who choose to adopt for reasons other than infertility), different paths can lead to motherhood. The most common of these is adoption.

If you decide adoption is for you, you are in good company. Most women who adopt are beyond thirty-five with a large percentage of those over forty. Some of them are pretty famous, including Diane Keaton, Marie Osmond, Jamie Lee Curtis, Rosie O'Donnell, Glenn Close, Mia Farrow, Donna Mills, Connie Chung and Sharon Stone.

Adoptive parents are not "lesser than" biological parents. Forming a family through adoption is not second best to being a "real" family. It *is* a real family. The love that flows between a child and his parents is as unequivocally strong through adoption as it is through biology.

Ask any woman who has done both: "When people ask me which one is my 'real' child, I have to stop and think, 'What are they talking about?'" says one forty-five-year-old author and mother of four: three adopted, one biological.

The more I meet adoptive mothers, the more I realize what a wide spectrum of adoption experiences are possible. There are several avenues one can take to becoming an adoptive mother: There is no definitely right, absolutely wrong or unconditionally best way to adopt. What is okay for you (an interracial child?) may not be okay for a friend (an open adoption?). Twelve women trading stories over coffee recently prove it: Though the outcome was the same (the adoption of a very wanted child), no two of the experiences that got them there were alike.

This chapter offers generic information about the adoption process. It is *impossible* to cover every detail of every form you will be asked to fill out for every type of adoption there is, since a world of variables exist. Other resources dedicated strictly to adoption—books, magazines, online sites, your local adoption agencies, friends—will fill you in once you decide which way you want to go.

What this chapter will do is define the basic types of

adoption available, outlining what is common to each type.

Most future adoptive mothers worry about how they'll know if they are getting the "right" child. When I worried over this, I was told by adoptive mothers before me that the right child will find his or her way home to us. Now that I stand on the other side of the experience, I have no doubt this is true; the more I watch adoptive mothers with their children, the more I am amazed that they found each other.

Trust your inner voice, for it will tell you what turns to make so that you can find the child you were meant to parent. The morning my husband, Jules, and I were to let our agency know if we wanted to accept Skyler or not—based on a one-minute video, a fuzzy photo and an even fuzzier sketch of his medical history—we went for a walk to talk it through. We happened to have his paperwork with us. I had barely read it because I was so overwhelmed by the prospect of *that* child in *that* photo possibly living under my roof and under my care.

We glanced at the papers as we walked and talked. My husband suddenly stopped. "Omigod!" he said. "Did you read what date his birthday is?" I hadn't. "It's October twentieth." This was incredibly serendipitous. My husband's birthday is October twenty-second. Mine is October twenty-seventh.

Before we had a chance to fully react to that news, I looked at my feet where someone had dropped a watch. The time read 7:11, the two traditional numbers of luck . . .

222 ♥ Getting to Mommyhood

what tellers of fortune these coincidences turned out to be for us! Skyler is the perfect completion to our family unit.

If you choose to go through the adoption process, trust that your inner voices will speak to you just as they have spoken to tens of thousands of other adoptive mothers who can't imagine their lives without their adopted children in them.

First Things First: Letting Go of the Old, Greeting the New, Grieving the Loss of Fertility

If you have gone through infertility treatments with all the accompanying emotional ups and downs, hopes and disappointments that come each cycle, you are well advised to clear out any residual grief you have about the loss of the ability to have your own biological child before you adopt. Why? For several reasons.

The first is that adoption also has lots of twists and turns. It is going to require your full attention and enthusiasm. More importantly, if you are harboring any leftover resentment about "having" to adopt rather than having your "own" child, your adopted child will know it. Your ability to form a warm mother–child bond will be inhibited and perhaps devastated throughout your entire mothering lifetime. This obviously benefits no one.

This kind of resentment can turn into distrust of the

child. One couple adopted a five-month-old child whom, when taken to the beach, crawled over to a stranger's blanket and sat himself down, perfectly content. Instead of thinking how cute he was to do that, the adoptive parents—who had not gotten over the fact that they could not have a biological child—accused the child of having attachment disorder as a result of this one incident; whatever the child did from that moment on, the parents were poised to pounce on him as not being good enough, no matter how trumped up or ridiculous the charge.

They ignored their own grief of infertility and therefore viewed their new child through a cloud of prejudice.

Other Older Adoptive Moms

Other adoptive moms you will meet can tell you what feelings they experienced. Anxiety is certainly not out of the question, but excitement should also be a big part of it, not dread or depression because you will be an adoptive mother, not a biological one.

One mother who had spent four years in fertility treatments before choosing to adopt sums it up this way: "Yes, I was disappointed that I couldn't get pregnant. But the bottom line was I wanted to be a mother, not a baby producer. I picked myself up, found out what I needed to do to adopt, and got on with it. And now I have a beautiful child to love and I can't remember those old feelings of disappointment. Coming home to her every day—isn't that what it's all about?"

Another important piece of advice adoptive mothers pass on is to be aware that there are many variables within the many variables of adoption. In other words, each agency or facilitator will have its own policies. Then, in addition, each type of adoption also has its rules. As you go through the process, keep in mind that whichever type you settle on, do not feel locked in by the particular agency's rules (they are only the final word on what their agency requires, not what the state or country requires). You do not want to take a child into your home under circumstances you feel uncomfortable with.

Advocate for yourself at every turn.

Common Fears About Adoption (And Some Assurances)

- **"The birth mother will take my child back"**: This is the most common fear amongst women adopting. It's also the biggest of myths surrounding adoption. Most adoptions last a lifetime between happy adoptive parents and wonderful adopted children of all ages and all races. While images of a screaming baby being returned to his "real" mother may be interesting stuff to watch on TV, the chances of this scenario happening in your life are very, very, *very* slim.

Not one person I spoke with reported of a child reclaimed by the birth mother after the child was living with the adoptive mother, or knew of anyone who had—and that includes agencies and facilitators, as well as lawyers who handle adoptions. This is not to say that occasionally a birth mother will change her mind before the baby is relinquished to you; hopefully, the birth mother you choose will get counseling throughout her pregnancy so this will never be a concern. Even more rarely does one hear about adoption "scams."

One more thing: Since international adoptions most often prohibit a child to be matched with prospective parents until the birth parents' rights have been severed, a birth mother reclaiming an internationally adopted child is extremely difficult to accomplish. So, if this is a real concern for you, you might want to consider this type of adoption.

- **The process takes too long:** Some forms of adoption take longer than others. Some agencies or facilitators will also take longer than others. One woman we spoke with took two years to get her son because of several "failed" adoptions (usually meaning birth mothers who changed their minds before the baby was born). Another couple took a quick six months to get an infant in their own state; another spent the same amount of time adopting a child overseas. This is an important point to check (via references) with the agency, facilitator or country or state of your choice.

- **The process is too expensive:** Adoption, depending on the avenue you choose, can cost from zero to thirty-five thousand dollars or more. In some cases, you may even get a subsidy for adopting a special-needs child. (See the Nuts and Bolts section of this chapter for a range of fees according to the type of adoption.)

  It is also important to keep in mind that you do not have to pay all the fees in one lump-sum up front. You pay piecemeal throughout the process. The costs can sometimes be borrowed; also, always check with your business or church to inquire if they offer financial assistance. Some offer several thousand dollars to help you complete your adoption (Wendy's restaurants, founded by the late Dave Thomas, himself an adoptee who was a very vocal adoption advocate, offers four thousand dollars to each employee who is adopting and six thousand dollars if adopting a special needs child).

- **How can I love another woman's child?** The child you get through adoption will be yours just as surely as the child you might have gotten through a petri dish or the regular "homemade" way. Besides, children come with their own agenda, whether or not they come with your DNA. Take comfort in the knowledge that a child's outcome is thought to be half environmental (that's the part you will affect for the better) and half genetics. Go back and read the definition of what a mother is. The woman who gave birth to your child is a woman to be blessed for sure. You and she have an unwritten contract whether or not you ever met her: She did the part you couldn't (get pregnant), and you are doing the part she couldn't (raise, love, discipline, play with, teach, kiss, care for, feed, do homework with, change diapers of, clothe, sing with, take roller-skating, stay up all night with when sick, read to, give birthday parties for, hug, cook for, your child).

"I am not sorry that we did not have our own biological child. This is the child who was meant for us. She just came to us in a different way from what I expected," a happy forty-four-year-old mother of an adopted two-year-old told us. "But I know she is the child I am supposed to mother."

If these feelings that you cannot love "another woman's child" persists throughout the adoption process, you might be wise to seek counseling and also consider becoming a mother another way.

- **What if my child would rather live with his birth mother?** The National Council for Adoption believes that much of what is written about an adopted child having a need to find his or her birth parents is quite exaggerated. In fact, it turns out that the majority of children who grow up adopted do not have a hunger to track down their biological parents or overthrow their adoptive parents in favor of a relationship with their biological parents.

That said, if you are adopting an older child who has memories of his or her home life before coming to live with you—a home life this child possibly misses out of guilt now that his or her life has improved under your roof—you can guide this child through and forge a new closeness with you as a result. "The history is there. The child's life did not start when he moved in with you," reminds a spokesperson for the National Adoption Center.

If you are adopting an infant or very young child, early memories of life before you will be murky, if they exist at all. The connection your child will have with his or her biological parents growing up will depend on the type of adoption you choose. (See the Nuts and Bolts section of this chapter.)

- **What if I fail the home study?** Not likely. First of all, home studies have a reputation for having barks worse than their bites—barring skeletons in your closet (such as a record of child abuse—but why would you be reading this book if you had one?). Regardless of whether or you rent or own, live in a mansion or an apartment, make a lot of money or don't have much left over after the bills, you will get the same equal shot at "passing" a home study.

Home-study agencies are licensed by the government. In the very unlikely event you do "fail," you can appeal to the regulating agency or even try another home study agency.

Read the section on home studies further along in this chapter.

A Roller Coaster of Emotions

If I had a dollar for every time I was patted on the head while simultaneously being pacified with the statement, "Adoption is a leap of faith," I would have had enough money to pay for my son's adoption. What else could it be but a leap of faith when you hand over money to complete strangers who tell you that out of the millions of children in the universe, they will find the exact right child for you? And while you are waiting for this happy moment, you must fill out, notarize and *re*-notarize piles of seemingly superfluous and supercilious paperwork! "And all because my hormones didn't work right!" as one infertile forty-three-year-old adoptive mother summed up. It's a roller coaster of emotions.

Is adoption any more of a roller coaster than infertility treatments or waiting to give birth? Only those who have been through both would venture to say—and even they can't say for sure, since some adoptions are easier to live through than some pregnancies and vice versa.

Rare is the adoption that has no bumps on the trail. But when the climb is over and you are at the end of the trail with your precious child in tow, any tribulations will seem small and far removed. They will become part of your common family history to be retold on each family anniversary ("Mommy, tell me about when you and Daddy came to bring me home.").

"Adoptive" Mother Defined

Adoptive mothers are not glorified babysitters who do the work until the "real" mother shows up. Adoptive mothers *are* the real mothers (change a few diapers, clean some spit-up off your best blouse or hear your child say, "You are my best friend" and try to deny you aren't).

"I was afraid that my child would turn to me one day and say, 'My real mother would never make me do so much homework . . . My real mother would let me drive the car . . . My real mother would let me put a ring through my nose . . .'" one adoptive forty-seven-year-old mother of a two-year-old best summed it up. "Then I started thinking about what it meant to be a 'real' mother and I realized that that's me. It's me who is there when he is sick, when he needs help with his homework, when anything goes on with his life. I'm the one who is always here. What is a mother if not that?"

Breastfeeding (Yes!) Your Adopted Infant

If you feel a need to breastfeed your newly adopted new-born, rest assured it is not some pie-in-the-sky dream. While it may not be easy or as fruitful as you hope (but breastfeeding a child you gave birth to can also be a struggle at first), devices can be purchased that will aid you in stimulating your own breast milk, so that you may breastfeed your child. Contact a local obstetrician or pediatrician or look in the phone book for a lactation consultant or a La Leche League chapter close to you.

Telling Your Child

Not telling your child the true facts of his or her life is crazy-making, since children can usually feel when someone is hiding a secret from them. They are very intuitive creatures. On the contrary, telling your child about how you became a family is a wonderful and comforting experience for you and your child. Once your child starts asking questions, keep his or her age in mind when you answer. What is it your child really wants to know? Here are three anecdotes that might help you keep a perspective:

1. We never kept his adoption a secret from Skyler, though when he was a toddler, we weren't sure what it meant to him. So when he and I were driving home

one night, he asked, "Mommy, where did I come from?" I thought to myself, *"Uh oh. Here comes the 'Did-I-come-from-your-tummy' question."*

I decided to see where he wanted to take this by saying, "Mommy comes from New York. Do you remember where you came from?" "Oh yes," he deadpanned. "I came from Rite-Aid."

It took me a moment to realize that we had just come from the mall—and the Rite-Aid drugstore in particular.

2. At his preschool, three-and-a-half-year-old adopted Trevor saw many of his classmates' pregnant mothers. "Mommy, did I come from your tummy?" he asked his forty-eight-year-old mother. "You came from my heart," she responded. This delighted Trevor; he could see exactly what she meant, for right over her heart is a freckle that he believed was the healed-up hole he came out of.

3. A seven-year-old girl wanted to know if she came from her adoptive forty-two-year-old mother's tummy. After an age-appropriate discussion about how babies are formed that probably droned on too long for the child's attention span, the girl said she only wanted to know if she came from her mother's tummy because she was trying to figure out if she was a human or a bird!

I repeat: Try to find out what your child wants to know

before answering this sensitive question; it's probably more sensitive for you than for he or she.

Telling Others

Adoption is a personal family matter. This should not be misconstrued to mean that adoption is something to be ashamed of. It is personal business that involves your child, a child who most likely will be too young to give you a well thought-out response to whether or not he or she wants to share the facts of his birth—and with whom—until he or she is much older.

Certainly most adoptive parents share this information with close friends and family at the very minimum. Others opt to tell everyone they meet, while some wear it as a badge. Still others, albeit a small minority, keep it to themselves because they worry about some unenlightened segments of society continuing to put a stigma on adoption.

"When the media kept referring to President Reagan's adult son as 'his adopted son, Michael,' I thought to myself it sounded belittling. Why would I want that label on my son for the rest of his life?" one fifty-three-year-old adoptive mother of a five-year-old boy confessed.

On the flip side, well-intentioned but uninformed people will often tell adoptive parents how "nice" it was of them to "take" an "unwanted" child. Typically an adoptive parents' reaction mirrors this mother's: "I didn't adopt a child to be altruistic. I did it for *me* because I wanted to be a mother. The fact that it was going to benefit a child who was unwanted or uncared for by her birth parents was just a by-product."

The facts of how your child came into your life should neither be a dark secret nor a topic to be discussed every day. It is my experience that most adoptive families settle comfortably into a middle ground and treat their family as a flawless whole.

Creating New Family Traditions: Celebrating Family Anniversary or Adoption Day

In our home, we celebrate an annual family anniversary; in our view we became a family on the date Skyler's adoption became final.

We keep the celebration intimate and simple by buying a family present like a board game we can all play together or a music CD we'd all enjoy, followed by dinner out at a family-friendly restaurant.

Referring to yourselves as an "adoptive family" means that your child is on par with everyone else in the family, especially the other kids who may be biological. An adoption happens to the whole family, not to the adopted child alone.

What If Your Adopted Child's Culture Is Different from Yours?

As children with different cultures grow up, they generally react in two diametrically opposed ways to their birth culture, if it is different from their parents' or friends'. On the down side, they may reject learning or even acknowledging their original culture: One possibility is that it may include painful memories. On the other end of the spectrum, there are those children who want to dress, eat and speak and live their native culture.

As adoptive parents, no matter how your child reacts to his or her culture, keep mementos for your child while he or she is growing up. You can collect trinkets, newspaper articles, music and books, as well as subscribe to magazines. Try forming a playgroup of children adopted from the same culture as your child's. Help your child find out as much about his or her culture of origin as he or she would like to know.

Types of Adoptions:
The Nuts and Bolts

Open Adoptions

Formal open adoptions as the standard for adoptions within the United States are a relatively new phenomenon within the last two or so decades. Open adoption means that the adoptive parents and the birth parents agree on how much contact everyone will have through the child's life. The amount of contact varies from adoption to adoption; settling it in advance affords all adult parties the right to say what they will, and won't, agree to. As with anything else that involves humans and human emotions, the experiences and possibilities vary widely. Some adoptive parents enjoy and encourage a close bond with the birth parents and birth siblings; still other adoptive parents find it discomforting to so much as send an annual letter and updated photo.

Birth parents likewise vary in how much contact they want with the child. Some may not want to attend birthday parties or have any reminders of the child, once he or she is born and handed over. For these mothers, knowing that their biological child is being loved and brought up in a great home can be enough.

In open adoption, the prospective adoptive parents are chosen by the birth mother (or birth parents if the birth father is present in the birth mother's life). These adoptions are arranged privately or through social agencies. Generally, the birth parents' rights are not relinquished until after the child has been placed.

Open adoptions generally come with a good history about the birth child and birth family, which is viewed by open-adoption advocates as a big plus. (Closed adoptions generally do not have a lot of information to pass on.)

Open domestic adoption can occur in two basic ways:

Domestic Public Adoption

Open adoptions that are run by public governmental agencies are the least expensive way to go. They generally cost between zero and twenty-five hundred dollars. While the financial aspects are clearly affordable, this form of adoption can take a long time, since potential parents work through the foster-adopt system.

Children are separated from their birth parents for a variety of reasons. Each situation, however, boils down to one thing: the birth parents are unable to care for their children in a manner agencies charged with their welfare deem appropriate. (*Note:* This does not include newborns voluntarily given up through private adoptions.) In public adoption, you work directly with a caseworker to select a child; you do not choose a birth mother yourself.

Once taken from their biological parents, children are put into the foster care system, whose primary goal is to try to reunite the child with his or her parents, not put the child up for adoption. If the court is satisfied that reuniting is not possible (which can take years), the child at last becomes available for adoption. In the meantime, however, the child has been in foster homes where the foster parents may or may not want to adopt him or her. If not, the child is then offered to other potential adoptive parents on a sort of first-come, first-served basis.

The advantage to a public open adoption is that you get to know a child during the processing. Public agencies work slowly, sometimes frustratingly so; as the potential adoptive parents, you will meet the child in a chaperoned environment and work toward being able to let him stay with you overnight.

This is a great choice, especially if you are interested in an older child, a special needs child, a sibling group or are not concerned about ethnic background. Over 100,000 children with a mean age of over five are available through public adoption (if you are interested in a younger child, be sure to let your caseworker know that). The length of time from start-up to welcoming a child into your home can vary widely—depending on what age, etc. you are looking for and on how much work needs to be done on the child's paperwork.

Domestic Private Adoption

These adoptions can run ten thousand dollars upwards to thirty-five thousand dollars or more. Legal fees, governmental agency payments (even though the adoption is private, it must still conform to legal requirements), adoption service providers, interstate costs if they apply, as well as payments for the medical and basic living costs of the birth mother are some of the expenses that add up. This latter expense can vary widely depending on what month of the birth mother's pregnancy you enter the picture. These fees—as any adoption fees—are not paid in one lump-sum but rather over a period of time, some even after your child is home with you.

Private adoptions are completed either through an adoption lawyer, an adoption facilitator (who probably works with a lawyer) or a private agency that will connect you with a birth mother and walk you through the paperwork you need to complete. As potential domestic open-adoptive parents, you will be asked to put together a portfolio—photos, letters, in essence a resume of who you are—so facilitators can "introduce" you to prospective birth mothers. Typically, the birth mother chooses the parents of her child in this way, whether it is arranged through an intermediary or directly.

In addition, obstetricians and ads placed by either the birth parents or prospective adoptive parents can be a source of reliable contacts: Finding a child through ads in newspapers is a legally utilized method allowed in many places. Even if you do not live in one of these places, you may either answer ads from areas where this is legal or place ads where they are allowed; in either case, you will want to use a lawyer to make sure your agreement with the birth mother is legal.

The time frame to complete an independent adoption is generally less than through public agencies; acceptance criteria are also more relaxed. If you are interested in a newborn, domestic private adoption is for you: It is rare to find older children this way unless it is through a family arrangement.

One drawback to this method is that the risk of the mother changing her mind, while still very small, most often happens with private open adoption. For this reason, it is advisable to stress that you want the birth mother to go through counseling while she is pregnant and after she gives birth. This will add a measure of assurance that the birth mother won't want to reclaim the child.

One other cautionary note: Before you sign any contracts, make sure the agency or other go-between you choose is licensed to act as an adoption facilitator.

International Adoptions

Americans adopt more children from foreign countries than any other nation on earth (there are 300,000 children in Russian orphanages alone). The numbers of internationally adopted children rose from 8,000 in 1980 to over 15,000 by the end of the 1990s. International fees can end in the highest ranges of adoption, running from fifteen thousand to thirty-five thousand dollars or more. As with private open adoption, payments to facilitators, government and in-country agencies are spread out over the length of the adoption process.

Not all foreign countries allow international adoption at all times: In other words, even if a country is known for allowing adoption by foreigners, it might not allow it at the time you are interested in adopting from there. If you are not sure if the country you are interested in is available, you can find out in one of several ways:

- Call the local foreign consulate of the country(ies) you are interested in.

- Speak to agencies that work internationally. Keep in mind, however, that an agency that specializes in China does not necessarily have contacts—or many contacts—for Russian adoptions.

- Read current issues of adoption magazines. The ads in these publications are a bounty of information.

- Ask friends, family and coworkers if they know anyone who has adopted internationally.

In many cases, adopting internationally means a shorter waiting period as well as a wider age range of available children than private open adoption completed domestically. In addition, most foreign adoptions take place after the birth mother has relinquished her rights to the child, which means the chances of the child being reclaimed are practically nonexistent. The adoption becomes final when the adoptive parents come in-country to pick their child up. It also means that these adoptions are closed: There is rarely contact with the birth parents after your child is home with you. Since international adoptions are most often closed, the manner in which adoptive parents are matched with a child switches from being chosen by birth parents (as in private domestic adoption) to choosing a child through your facilitator. One downside of international adoption is that the medical and family history may not be very complete, though this varies.

Most children available from foreign countries have spent at least some of their lives in orphanages. Orphanages can vary widely in care not only from country to country, but from region to region within the same country. In the majority of these cases, the children get the best care possible despite media reports to the contrary. The media is in the business of entertaining: The truth of the mundane day-to-day in most orphanages would bore viewers. But it behooves you to check out the orphanage you'll be dealing with by getting references from other adoptive families who have been there. Choose a facilitator who works with orphanages that get high marks from those who have seen them firsthand.

When the time comes to bring your child home, go to the orphanage yourself, where possible, rather than have someone deliver her to an airport near your home. This may be your only chance to see firsthand where your child came from; as a result, you may be your child's only source of information as he asks questions about what his country or village was like when he left it.

After having made the decision to adopt out of country, you will work with a facilitator who can advise you about the different countries open for adoption at the time. The facilitator will either make all arrangements for you, including in-country travel and boarding, or will be there only to offer guidance as to what steps you need to take next. While the former may charge more, it will be to your advantage to go with the agency that shoulders most of the work, since finding your own way through the maze of your own country's paperwork is difficult enough without having to do it in a foreign country as well.

In addition to working with an adoption facilitator or private agency, international adoptions can also be completed with the aid of a lawyer who specializes in them, though the numbers of international adoptions completed in this manner are smaller.

Getting Started

Once you start telling everyone you know that you are thinking about adopting, you will be amazed at how many people have experience with it—if not personally, through family members or friends. Talk to as many people who have adopted as you can; rare is the adoptive mother who is not thrilled to tell you honestly about her experience, to recommend an agency or even invite you to meet her kids.

Turn also to adoption magazines; the articles, editorials, opinions and ads are a wealth of information about facilitators and the process in general. Amass brochures from the agencies that appeal to you so you get an idea of how each works. Ask to be invited to their annual picnics where you can meet the children they have helped match to adoptive parents. It's a great opportunity to learn about the procedure as well as meet firsthand real live adopted kids. Ask the new parents how long their adoption took and if it was close to the time the agency had estimated for them.

Check your local yellow pages for adoption agencies while keeping in mind that you do not have to use a local facilitator. Read parenting publications and local newspapers for announcements of introductory talks on adoption.

Once you choose an agency, lawyer or facilitator, get an *up-front* estimate of fees and what the schedule for payments will be. How will the facilitator match you with a referral for a child—through personal contact (as in the case of domestic adoption) or via photos and videos, which is most frequently used in international adoption? What is the timeline you will have to decide on a referral?

How many resources for children does your facilitator

work with? This is important because it can affect how long your process will take: the more contacts, the more referrals. Does the staff answer your questions in a timely manner?

If a restriction is put on you by the agency that you are not comfortable with, ferret out if it is the agency's policy versus governmental regulation. I learned to do this the hard way: One agency told me that I was too old to adopt a child under ten years old from Russia. As a result, I came this close to giving up the idea of adoption. I later discovered that this was that agency's policy, not Russia's. I found another agency to work with.

I cannot stress how important it is to do your homework before you sign on the dotted line. Check out the adoption resources listed in the resource chapter of this book. In addition to reading everything you can about the various types of adoption, there are an enormous number of Web sites manned (or wo-manned) by adoptive parents and facilitators. While these sites can be a hotbed of unfounded rumors, they can also be a great resource of information and handholding.

The Home Study

A local home study is completed no matter where you are adopting your child from—including internationally— or what type of adoption you are pursuing.

Ostensibly, a home study is conducted to evaluate you as

a prospective parent to let the governing agency know what a terrific mother you will be. It satisfies a government request and is just one of many pieces of paper that must have all the i's dotted and t's crossed in order to bring your adoption to a legally binding close.

The agency you hire to conduct your home study will send a licensed home study caseworker to interview you, your partner and any other household members, such as other children living at home. The caseworker will look over your home, and depending on the governing agency's policies, might ask you to make some changes to comply with their rules, e.g., putting safety locks on all your drawers and cabinets. Some requests may seem out of hand to you: One couple was asked to put safety locks on cabinets on behalf of the ten-year-old child they were adopting.

The interviews will take place over three or four visits (not all of them need to be in your home) and could take two months or more. If you are adopting internationally, the process will be completed before you get your child (though some follow-up may be done just for record-keeping purposes). If you are adopting domestically, the home study frequently is not completed until after the child is living in your home. This is another way domestic and international adoptions are different.

If you have not already made up your mind about what method of adoption you will use, your caseworker can give you his or her perspective on the pros and cons of each type.

Hints on "Passing"

Your caseworker and the resultant report she will write are a key part in getting your file completed so you can complete the adoption process. As stated earlier in this chapter, your chances of "failing" your home study are pretty small. Remain calm, be thoughtful in your answers, cooperate with reasonable requests (e.g., gathering photos for the report) and remember that you have a right to feel comfortable with who has been assigned to your case. If you are not, request another worker. "I was really concerned about passing the home study. If I had known how relaxed our social worker would be with us, I never would have lost sleep over it," says an adoptive forty-eight-year-old mom of three.

There is no one-size-fits-all home study good for every circumstance; however, certain standard topics must be covered in order to satisfy the governing agency. Your goal is to get those questions answered efficiently and to the point, then get the caseworker to write the report in a timely manner so you can move on to the next steps. When it is finally completed, check the home study over personally (as you should with all your paperwork) to look for errors. Our caseworker, albeit a sweetheart of a woman, made at least three glaringly visible errors, including dates of crucial events.

The home study agency and the facilitator will often be two separate agencies; inquire to see if your facilitator approves of the home study agency you want to use. Your facilitator can recommend a home study agency that will do the best job for the type of adoption you are looking toward.

Typical Questions (And Answers)

Your home study caseworker will ask questions about your health, finances, daily life and your relationships. It is unnecessary for you to answer questions that you deem too personal. One agency we considered sent us an introductory questionnaire that contained questions about our sex life. Stunned, we could not get a satisfactory answer as to why they needed that information. Subsequently, the next three agencies we considered assured us that we did not need to answer humiliating questions in order to adopt. We hired one of those agencies instead.

Those kinds of questions aside, it will be to your advantage to thoroughly answer questions about your relationship and home life that build up your lifestyle: e.g., "We love to go to amusement parks"; "We have brothers and sisters who can't wait to become aunts and uncles"; "My husband will make a great daddy, because he always listens to my problems."

At some point, it is likely you will be asked to get fingerprints. These will be run through child abuse and criminal records.

Special Concerns

- **Age Limits:** There is no across-the-board legal age limit to adoption. Some agencies or facilitators (including private lawyers) may have their own cap on what age the adoptive mother must be in order for them to work with you. This may also be true if you are adopting out of the country: Some countries are mostly interested in older mothers (like China), while others won't allow anyone over a certain age. In international adoption, in particular, it is the mother's age that is regarded. Many countries still believe that it is the mother who does all the parenting, and therefore Dad's age doesn't count as heavily.

- **Single Parenting:** There are no regulations that broadly prohibit single-mother adoption, whether it be domestic, private, foreign, open or closed. However, it is your responsibility to thoroughly check out policies and laws before you plunk your money down to a specific facilitator who promises you a carefree adoption.

CHAPTER 14

A Few Words About Foster Mothering

In 1988, 340,000 American children were in foster care; just ten years later, the numbers crept up by another 200,000. The children in foster care range in age from infancy through their teens and are almost evenly divided by race across the board.

The mean age of a foster child is nine-and-a-half years old with about 21,000 under the age of one. The mean time a child resides in a foster home is between two and three years.

What Is a Foster Mother?

A foster mother is the state or county government-appointed *temporary* guardian of a child who is in the foster care system and who is in need of a home. The idea of foster care is to fill a gap—get the kids to school, to the dentist, help with their homework, celebrate their birthdays—in short, do everything you would do for your own legal child—until such time the parents can reenter the picture or a court decides a permanent adoptive home should be found for the child.

"Becoming a foster mother does not mean that the mother will mother the child for a lifetime," explained one fifty-eight-year-old foster mother online. "I had three bio kids of my own (ten, eleven and fifteen), when I decided to become a foster mother. I just saw so many kids in need, how could I not? My own kids have always had a say about which kids come to live with us."

Who Qualifies As a Foster Mother?

According to the National Foster Parent Association, a foster mother can be an adult woman of any age and may rent or own her home as long as there is room for a foster child in it. The mother may also work outside of the home and the family must be able to take care of their own financial needs sans the income from foster care.

Each state has its own spin on requirements, but generally you will undergo a home study similar to the one adoptive parents must go through, as well as be fingerprinted, interviewed and trained.

What Does a Foster Mother Do?

In addition to everyday responsibilities, a foster mother must work with the different agencies that are legally responsible for the child. This will include visits with the caseworker to make plans for the child.

Duties could also include making sure that the child gets to visit with his or her sometimes-difficult parents; this event can leave the child feeling very emotional. It can be a challenge for the foster mother to hold her tongue in these situations: "We need to have respect for the bio parents. There, but for the grace of God, go I. If you degrade the bio parent to the child, you are degrading the child, too," reports another foster mom.

Rights of Foster Mothers

As a foster mother, you will have the right to:

• Refuse any placement you are offered based on criteria of your choice—such as the age of the child.

• Ask that the child be removed from your home if the placement becomes too difficult for you.

Is Foster Parenting Like Tryout Mothering?

Some women believe they will "try out" parenting by becoming a foster mother before they decide whether or not to have kids on a permanent basis. For obvious reasons, this isn't a good idea: Temporary care of a child in an emergency situation, who you do not have legal custody of, *is not the same* as caring for a child who will be in your home and in your life for the rest of your life.

Remember, it is the primary purpose of foster care to reunite children with their parents.

However, if you would like to get a taste of foster parenting, you can volunteer for emergency foster care which usually lasts one month or less, until such time that a plan can be made for the child.

The Ups and Downs of Being a Foster Mother

- The children arrived in your care as the result of a crisis in their families: death, abuse, abandonment and a whole host of other not-so-good reasons. They were likely taken from their homes by court order, followed possibly by a police officer arriving to physically remove them.

- It can be very trying being the interim parent; making

it more discomforting, you probably won't know at the outset how long the "interim" will last.

- Letting go becomes a big part of your vocabulary; you especially need to let go when you are preparing the child to move on to a situation that you might not approve of . . .

- . . . However, it is so rewarding to be there as a safety net—a loving safety net—for a child who is hurt (physically and/or emotionally) and in need.

- While about 100,000 children in foster care are available for adoption on any given day, don't count on foster care as a road to adoption. It is not automatic that because you are the foster parent, you are first in line to adopt the child you are foster parenting at the moment. If adoption is what you are really after, you must be very clear with the agency you are working with right from the beginning.

- Perhaps the biggest plus was summed up by one forty-eight-year-old foster mom: "The biggest pleasure is to see a child with self-confidence where there was none before."

Rumors of Rewards

While a fee is paid to the foster parent to cover a part of the basics—food, shelter, clothing—this is no get-rich-quick scheme. A foster mother has to be committed not only to the mothering duties, but to also taking money out of her own pocket for some of the extras that the small fee paid does not cover.

. . . And the Real Reward

The real reward is the everyday fact of having these children in your home. "People tell me how great I am for taking in foster children. But I'm the lucky one. They have brought me such joy," an over-forty foster mom says.

PART FOUR

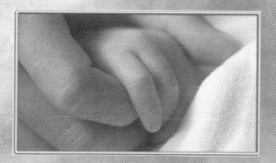

Life Goes On

CHAPTER 15

In It for the Long Haul: Taking Care of Yourself for the Sake of Your Child

Draw your child close to you, feel the velvet that is his cheek or the warmth of her head as she snuggles on your lap.

I defy you to come up with a better reason to take care of yourself.

And not just at the beginning when you are swept away by your dreams of what you want for you and your child—but over all the years as the dreams shift and reality settles into day-to-day living.

Becoming a mother means you are in it for the long haul. You are given a great opportunity to reevaluate how you care for yourself; then make the changes needed so that your future has as healthy a foundation as possible.

Now is the time to commit to a healthy rest-of-your-life.

Staying Motivated

If you are "typical" of women who become mothers later on, most likely you will not find it too hard to stay motivated. Just by the mere fact that you'll have a twenty-four-hour-per-day perpetual motion machine in your house for the next eighteen or so years will keep you on the move.

If motivation to keep fit starts to wane, look at the alternative. It is a known fact that people who exercise are more likely to live a better quality of life. This is all well and good on its own, but when you think of it in terms of the future of your child, then taking care of yourself becomes an all-important priority. You will want to be able to enjoy your child in every way and on every level—that might mean hiking, practicing soccer, even being there to hold your own grandchild!

Keep a mental picture of yourself at your child's college graduation, at his or her wedding or playing with your grandchild.

There's your motivation.

Your Brain: Use It or Lose It

Even if you are a Rhodes Scholar, nothing will challenge you more than coming up with answers for your child's off-the-cuff and constant stream-of-consciousness questions.

As part of nature's course, the brain function starts to diminish as the years pass. This doesn't mean you are about to fall into premature senility; however, just like with other body parts, the brain needs to be exercised to stay fit. That way, you'll have a ready response when your child comes out of left field from his curious world with, "Mommy, why don't animals talk?"

Here are some simple ways to keep your mind sharp:

- Do demanding mental activities. Pencil-and-paper word games like crossword puzzles, word jumbles or seek and search are some examples. Often in magazine form, buy some to keep on your nightstand and in your baby bag. Do them as your little one digs in the sand at the park.

- Supplements like gingko biloba and vitamin E are good for the brain.

- Read challenging books and magazines (parenting topics, of course, but other interests as well). Read a newspaper every day, even if you only have time for the front page. Join a book club or a political club where you can discuss what you read.

- Write in a journal each day. Not only will this help keep your wordsmithing skills sharp, it'll be a great keepsake for you and your child.

- Learn a new word each week.

- Get a babysitter and attend lectures or workshops on a regular basis on any topic that interests you.
- Have adult conversations as often as possible.

Stamina, or How Not to Feel Too Pooped to Pop

Defined as a combination of endurance, strength and vigor, stamina is a quality that makes up the foundation of all you will experience as a mother. It's what you want more of, not less of. This does not mean, however, that you have to bypass the urge to nap or be a couch potato every now and then (as if you'll have time!).

Diminishing stamina is part of what occurs as we get older, just like the above-mentioned brain power; as young as age twenty-five, our metabolism starts to slow .05 to 1 percent per year. As a result, it's harder to get weight off, which compounds a slowing of energy. In addition, women have the added stamina-thief to contend with known as menopause. Hormonal changes caused by menopause can cause sleepless nights for one thing; did you know that menopausal symptoms start to creep in as much as fifteen years before the actual menopause occurs?

The best thing you can do is give yourself permission to not have to do it all. Don't burn the candle at both ends. Nap when the kids do (instead of always being tempted to fold laundry or vacuum) or take time out whenever you can. When they no longer nap, arrange a safe play space for them, while you lie down with your feet up and a good magazine. When he was too old for the playpen and too young to be left alone, I would let Skyler play on the floor of my bedroom while I read for a little bit. Whatever works for you, work toward arranging as stress-free a schedule as possible. Stress is known to quicken the loss of stamina.

Of course, eating well (see the section on Nutrition in this chapter) only adds to the quality of your stamina.

After all is said and done, if you feel you have less stamina than what would be considered normal, get thee to a doctor and run through the appropriate tests.

Exercise

If you are active now, all you need to do is maintain a place in your schedule to continue getting exercise. Sounds simple enough, but it may require more creativity on your part than you are used to. If your time is squeezed between working and family, it will take extra effort; but the effort is important to make. My own first mother's group would meet at the gym, so the moms could work out while the kids played together in childcare. Most gyms and workout centers have fixed times for childcare, so you can work out. Getting a jogging stroller while your child is still in the stroller phase is a popular alternative to the gym, but even with a regular stroller, you can walk your neighborhood or mall.

Buy a pair of barbells and include weight lifting and resistance exercises in your regimen (what better weight-lifting exercise than toting your chunky bundle of joy with sopping wet diaper up, down and around?). Alternate aerobics, weight lifting and stretching throughout your week. Weight lifting should be done every other day to give your muscles a chance to rest in between.

Weight-*bearing* exercises are those that put stress on the bone, which helps build bone mass. These types of exercises include hiking, dancing, using the treadmill (which can also be aerobic), jogging, walking (ditto, ditto), climbing stairs and using the weight machines at the gym.

Keep in mind that *some* exercise is better than no exercise.

Sedentary?

If exercise is something you've thought about doing but somehow never quite get around to it, read one of the several good books that teach how to exercise with baby. While just carrying your baby with one arm and juggling the laundry bag under the other will get you up and off the couch, there are lots of other things you can do. Work out with other mothers, trek the mall with your child in the stroller on rainy days, buy a baby backpack and take a nature walk on weekends with other families.

Good news! If getting to the gym for a longer workout seems like a luxury, try working out in ten-minute spurts several times a day (like a quick jog up and down the stairs) and still reap great benefits. As the slogan says, just do it.

Nutrition: Being a Mother Will Force You to Eat Better

. . . if for no other reason than you will be eating your child's leftovers; leftovers that are pretty healthy, since what else would you serve your child but nutritious eats?

Water

Drink lots of water even if you do not have a taste for it; include also other healthy liquids such as herbal teas. If your new life is too busy to count up eight glasses of water every day, buy a small sport drink bottle and keep refilling it (with bottled water preferably), carrying it with you everywhere. Ask for water in restaurants (with lemon) instead of other beverages.

Herbs

Two good herbs to take for general women's health are dong quai and ginseng. If you are planning to get pregnant or are nursing, let your doctor know that you take these (or any other) herbs.

Tofu

Tofu and other soybean products are excellent because they have *phytohormones,* which are helpful as we age, as well as being a good source of calcium and protein. Can't stand the taste, you say? Tofu takes on the taste of whatever you put on it or cook it with; it can be scrambled with eggs, thrown into tomato sauce, blended into salad dressings and anything else your creative chef-ness can come up with. Soybeans come in many forms: the edamame bean, miso for use as soups, soymilk (experiment with brands since taste can vary). Lots of products are made with tofu today, since this food has become so well respected. Don't forget to offer soy dishes to *all* your family members.

Fats

Don't overlook fat altogether; just make certain you use good ones, such as olive oil. Stay away especially from products made with palm and coconut oil.

Vitamins

Include vitamins C, E and the B's in your everyday diet. Yes, supplements are great and easy to take, but it's also important to get your vitamins and minerals from actual foods. Many health-food stores sell charts that show what food sources each vitamin and mineral can be found in.

Calcium

Foods rich in calcium are important because as we get older, if we do not have enough calcium in our diet, our body will "steal" it from our bones. Obviously not a good thing, this weakens our bones making it not only harder to heal properly if we break one, but opens the door to osteoporosis. Good sources of calcium include dairy products (buy *real* yogurt with cultures in it; the ice cream store variety or some store-bought ones with too much sugar or custard should only be occasional treats), dark green leafy vegetables like spinach, tofu, salmon and sardines (especially when the bones are eaten).

Eating Styles

Regular meals with healthy snacks will help keep your energy up. Take in the majority of your protein from complex carbohydrate sources such as oatmeal: They supply a steady source of energy. Eat smaller "meals" more frequently for the same reason: a salad and soup for lunch, pasta and steamed vegetables for dinner. Use fruits for quick pick-me-ups as well as a healthy source of refreshing liquids. When you are out with the little ones, don't forget to pack enough snack foods for you as well. Things like dried fruits, baked pretzels and whole-corn tortilla chips are good choices for both of you, and will keep in the baby bag for a long while.

Menopause

In most cultures, women who have stopped menstruating are treated with the greatest of respect: Native American women are given a seat at the Council of Elders where tribal decisions are made. Menopause is a phase of a woman's life that means she has acquired great wisdom to pass on to others. As a woman who delayed motherhood, you will be using your acquired wisdom to guide your child; your child will have an advantage, because you are his or her mother.

The Menopause Cycle

As you know by now, a woman is born with all the eggs she will ever have. With each cycle, as well as through attrition, the eggs recede to the point that they are no longer capable of supporting a menstrual cycle. Enter menopause.

Being in menopause is defined as the stoppage of twelve menstrual cycles in a row; in other words, you are not in menopause until a whole year has passed without a menstrual period. This is nature's way of signaling the end of child*bearing* (not to be confused with child*rearing*). Too, with the new technology (see the chapter on Infertility), it is not even automatically the end of childbirth.

Typically, by the age of fifty-two, most women today have entered into menopause. This is an average; some thirty-seven-year-old women have stopped ovulation and an occasional fifty-five-year-old hasn't. About fifteen years before menstruation stops, a woman's menstrual cycle starts to go through subtle changes: It might not be as regular, as long, as strong. It may come twice a month or not at all for two months in a row. Peri-menopause is the term used for women in this stage, entering the beginning of the end. As the woman's eggs run out, the ovaries cease functioning to create the menstrual process.

Symptoms

The most often referred-to symptoms are hot flashes and their evil twin, night sweats; the latter is when you wake up sweaty-wet on the nights your partner is begging you to turn on the heat. Hot flashes are pretty much as they sound: With no warning, heat flashes radiate throughout your body (FYI: Another word for flash is *twinkle*).

These symptoms are a result of the body's effort to regulate its core temperature through this period of hormonal upheaval.

Other less-talked-about symptoms include a sense of urgency to urinate and variations in frequency as well as leaking urine, since bladder muscles weaken. Practice Kegel exercises to tighten and relax the vaginal muscles.

Some women also complain about vaginal dryness (regular orgasms help), irritability (who wouldn't be with all those hot flashes) and forgetfulness. I remember giggling as my mother searched all over the room for the eyeglasses that were "hiding" atop her head.

What can you do to help if you are not already in menopause? Relax and realize that every woman goes through it. It is not a disease; it is a natural, normal part of aging and a rite of passage. Billions of women before you have gotten through it; so will you.

If you want to be proactive, rely on the old standbys of exercise and good nutrition to keep menopausal symptoms under control. Get regular checkups and discuss the latest therapies with your doctor. Follow the suggestions for nutrition in this chapter.

Also, consult with a doctor and ob/gyn who specializes in women your age about general health considerations, including keeping up your strength, osteoporosis prevention and menopause.

The Necessities of Pampering Yourself

Pamper yourself as often as you can. While this statement does not have to translate to "eat more chocolate cake," it is intended to recognize the hardest working woman you know: you!

If You Don't Have a Spiritual Life, Get One

I can't stress enough the importance of keeping connected to a higher meaning of life. The secure feeling you get from an inner life will maintain you when the going gets tough—and there will be bumpy patches during your mothering career. Taking time every single day for your Inner Life (I call it "Inner Fitness") is as important as your physical fitness regimen. Whether or not you consider yourself an active member of a religious or spiritual practice, find five minutes, preferably at the beginning of each day, to read something inspirational, pray, meditate or otherwise spend time with a quiet mind. A calmer, more positive attitude will be yours as your day unfolds. You will also accomplish more and feel more productive as a result of your daily "time-out."

In the evenings, write down a minimum of three things each day that you are grateful for. They do not have to be big things ("I won the lottery!") but the everyday things that make up the goodness of your life ("My pillow is so comfortable.").

Saying thank-you out loud will help you appreciate what you have. And who knows, maybe some entity "up there" or "out there" or somewhere in between will hear it and give you more of what you like.

Getting Away from It All

Get to a spa. Get a baby-sitter in the middle of the day in the middle of the week and go on a long hike alone. Hire someone to play with your little one when you are home one evening. Use the time to prepare a really healthy gourmet dish complete with wine (if you are not breastfeeding). Set the table with pretty plates, napkins, tablecloth and candles. Use the good silver.

Give yourself a facial for dessert.

Time Alone with Other Adults

Reach into the recesses of your past life, B.B. (Before Baby), and the conversations you used to have with other adults: Back then, words "poop," "reading readiness" and "soccer" rarely made their way to the dinner table. There is a whole world out there aside from your little guy (albeit he is the center of it). While chances are many of your old friends from your B.B. life have been lost along the way, you'll have lots of opportunity to meet new ones. Go to a movie with "the girls," start a book club and meet during baby's nap time, treat yourself to a mom's night out monthly.

Time Alone with Your Partner

One day in the not-too-distant future, the children will be too busy to make collages with you, and you and your partner will be left *home alone* staring at each other over the remote control! "Hello, do I know you?" you'll ask.

In the 1950s, marriages were couple-centered; as the

century progressed, child-centered families were favored. Today, psychotherapists and common sense agree that balance is required. Arrange for a babysitter on a regular weekly basis. Go someplace where the two of you can talk and remember: "Oh, yeah, *that's* why we fell in love!"

I Know We Don't Need to Remind You, But . . .

Smoking, alcohol, illegal drugs (or overdoing prescription drugs), burning the candle at both ends, eating junk food as a steady diet, too much caffeine, lack of exercise and living a stressful life are not the means to the end you want for yourself and your family.

Replace old bad habits with new and satisfying ones that benefit and befit your new role. Watching your children grow, you'll be glad for your decision to do so.

CHAPTER 16

Not-So-Secret Thoughts of Later-in-Life Mommies

"Your social life is radically changed. Come to think of it, your whole life is radically changed."

J.E., 42, BOY 4, GIRL 18 MONTHS

"The best part is being the recipient of hugs and kisses and 'I love you, mommy.' The worst is the constant bickering."

M.L., 48, BOY AND GIRL, BOTH 4

"You have to be prepared to rise to the occasion and do things without anyone patting you on the back for it. It's just expected of you to do these extraordinary ordinary things every day without thanks, raises or bonuses."

A.S., BOY 5

"I would probably have thought I knew it all at twenty.
Now, at forty-three, I'm quite sure I don't.
There's a lot to learn about the art of parenting."

P.J., 43, BOY 6

"I'm not anxious for my children to grow up,
I just don't want to get any older."

M.N., BOYS 5 AND 14 MONTHS

"Anyone becoming a mother better dig down deep
and know this decision is right for her,
regardless of her age."

C.T., 52, WAITING TO ADOPT

"I'm never bored. There is never enough time.
We are always on the run: play groups, swim lessons, etc.
I'm always busy, but it's fun busy. I know I'm less stressed
spending time with my child than I was before."

J.F., 39, GIRLS 3 AND 1

"You have to like kids and want *to spend*
time with your children."

R.A., 37, GIRL 3½

"Watching and helping him grow has been the
best part of my life so far. I don't think
I will ever get tired of it."

K.D., 46, BOY 4

*"I don't do all those things with my child that
the books recommend. If I did, I'd have no time for
anything else, and I need that. I try not to feel guilty.
It's hard though when I hear about little Joey or Hannah
going to dance lessons, Spanish lessons and the beach
house every weekend. Will my child miss out?"*

R.D., 47, BOY 6, GIRL 4

*"We are saving for college, retirement and
helping to care for my mother-in-law all at once.
It's a lot to bite off and then have to chew. But we'd never
want to go back to life without our children."*

S.M., 52, BOY 7, GIRL 4

*"I went to a psychotherapist to see if
I was out of my mind for wanting a child at my age.
After we talked about what my life was like, that I was
stable, happy and all those kinds of things, we decided I
should go for it. 'If that's your dream,' she said, 'do it.'"*

E.B., 47, GIRL 18 MONTHS

*"I'm worried that as my kids get older and
compare me to other mothers who are much younger
that they'll think I look really old and be ashamed of me.
I always felt sorry for the kids whose old-looking parents
came to school. The kids looked so embarrassed."*

C.T., 53, BOYS 1 (TWINS) AND 8.

*"I feel sad that I didn't have a child
when my parents were younger, so they could have
enjoyed my child as a grandchild much like they did
with my sisters' kids—it's not just about me or
my husband or even my child."*

D.C., 55, BOY 5

*"Becoming a mother, especially later on,
is such a positive thing to do, because it is
showing that I have faith in my future.
Why else would I do it?"*

M.L., 48, BOY AND GIRL, BOTH 4

*"What matters is what values I give
this child, who she turns out to be in some part
thanks to my efforts—not how old I was
when I became a mother."*

L.F., 52, GIRL 7

*"I long for this baby more than
I ever longed for any man or job—
or anything else for that matter—
in my whole life."*

D.D., 36, TRYING TO CONCEIVE

*"Just laying my eyes on him every morning
makes all the difference in my life."*

T.C., 55, BOY 7

*"No one's kisses have, or ever will,
thrill me like his do!"*

D.K., 44, BOY 6

*"I'm more careful to keep up with
dyeing the gray out of my hair now that
I have a small child."*

E.B., 47, GIRL 18 MONTHS

*"I would never have believed that one of
the biggest rewards of motherhood at this stage in
my life would be that I have less focus on my career
and myself. What a blessing it is to not
think about myself so much."*

R.D., 47, BOY 6, GIRL 4

*"I knew I had arrived as a
real mother when my husband asked what
I'd like for my birthday and all I could
think of was a new stroller."*

B.S., 38, GIRL 2

*"I know this: You can't place a value on the feeling
I get when I look into my child's eyes.
Yes, there certainly are dirty diapers and sleepless
nights and we are always tired, but . . ."*

M.R., 42, GIRLS 5 AND 3½, BOY 1

*"There is no question that I am a better mother today
than I would have been in my twenties.
No question."*

C.T., 53, BOYS 1 (TWINS) AND 8

*"A second child? He wasn't planned for,
but I was thrilled thinking about him while we
were waiting for him to be born. Now that he's here,
as much as I love him, if I could have fast-forwarded to
today, no, I wouldn't have had a second child.
He misses out in every way."*

C.O., 45, BOYS 6 AND 2

"You must, you must, you must
find time for yourself."

L.P., 44, BOY 2½

*"The problems are magnified because of my age;
there are some things that are much more challenging.
But the rewards are also magnified because I'm older.
I appreciate the fact of my motherhood very deeply."*

F.T., 49, GIRLS 3 AND 1

*"Age is a matter of mind. If you don't mind,
it doesn't matter—at least when it comes to the
parenting aspect; trying to* get *pregnant and
then giving birth is a different story."*

R.D., 47, BOY 6, GIRL 4

*"I miss going out at night, working out
on a regular basis, going to the movies on the
spur of the moment. Actually, doing anything
on the spur of the moment."*

L.S., 48, BOY 5

*"Make sure your partner is there at least
50 percent of the time to help."*

L.A., BOYS 5 AND 18 MONTHS

*"None of the rewards of my life have
equaled parenting. When I look at her, I know
what having 'a full heart' means."*

R.W., 41, GIRL 9 MONTHS

*"Am I selfish? Will I be too feeble to go
to his high school graduation? I don't know;
what I do know is that because I love him so very much,
if I die while he's still young, I will be leaving him
with the greatest legacy: a happy childhood."*

M.A., 52, BOY 3

*"There are days when I think
I could have ten more; there are days I think,
what was I thinking to have one?"*

L.S., 42, GIRL 18 MONTHS

*"I always thought I had a really full life
between my job, the classes I took, my busy social life.
I never realized how empty my life was until my sons showed
up. I am not regretful, but if I had known,
I would have done it sooner."*

A.P., 46, TWIN BOYS 4

*"I have a renewed lease on life and, because of her,
I want to make something more of myself."*

R.A., 37, GIRL 18 MONTHS

*"I know I'm not alone in this when I say
that I don't love both my children equally. One 'belongs'
to my husband, the other is 'mine.' And I see this
dynamic in lots of families with midlife
mothers and more than one child."*

C.O., 45, BOYS 6 AND 2½

*"When I was depressed before, I couldn't shake
it easily. Now, my daughter makes me feel
so positive just by her being."*

C.C., 43, GIRL 18 MONTHS

*"You fall in love with your child every day.
Before you know it, you are hooked."*

S.K., 47, GIRL 6 MONTHS

*"As an older parent, I've had time to see what
would be best in parenting a child in this day and age.
I am definitely parenting differently
than my parents did."*

F.T., 49, GIRLS 3 AND 1

*"Hearing my baby's first cry in the delivery room
was the sweetest sound I ever heard."*

M.L., 47, GIRL 6 WEEKS

*"I think if I were in my twenties, I probably
would have been more competitive with my child
because of my own insecurities. I would have done a lot
of second-guessing my decisions and not have been
as grounded as I am now as a mother."*

P.J., 43, BOY 6

*"Most people who do not know me
have no clue as to how much older I really am.
I see a lot of women around my age who
look much younger than they are."*

W.B., 49, BOY 4

*"The worst part of motherhood is having
to be totally responsible for a whole human being.
The best part is the unexpected love you get."*

L.S., 48, BOY 5

"I can't imagine my family without him. I can't imagine him anyplace else except in my home as my son. I would not be complete without him."

K.D., 46, BOY 4

"I felt I had so much stored up ready to give to this child as an older mother. I was educated and ready to pass on good values and couldn't wait to spend time with him teaching him all sorts of things. Boy, was I ready!"

B.S., 38, GIRL 2

"How do we do it? I don't know. We just get up every day and do what we need to do. I was always a mother, so I don't know any differently. I'm a lot more relaxed this time around."

C.W., 48, SONS 4 AND 21, GRANDSON 2

"I love all the commotion in my house. I think privacy is overrated."

E.B., 47, GIRL 18 MONTHS

"I don't mind pinching pennies. My kids learn they can get along on less."

M.R., 42, GIRLS 5 AND 3½, BOY 1

"We're glad we didn't have another child. It's hard enough giving one the attention he needs."

A.S., 40, BOY 5

"This is the most important thing I've done in my life. Though I do miss being able to read the newspaper leisurely in bed on Sundays."

W.B., 49, BOY 4

"One good thing is that being older with a young child forces you to keep your brain sharp. I find I'm getting sharper as he gets older, not the reverse."

R.W., 41, BOY, 9 MONTHS

"It's a real trade-off. Physically it's harder when you are older, but I know I wouldn't have been mentally ready back in my twenties."

B.S., 38, GIRL 2

"If I Could Turn Back the Clock, . . ."

"I would have started at thirty-five, not forty-eight."

"If I had known how much fun I'd be having, without question I would have done this sooner."

"People don't understand the intense feelings of grief you can have as the result of infertility. I would have gotten counseling about it."

"I tried to do it all on my own as a new, older single mother. If I had to do it over, I'd make sure I had some help, especially at the beginning."

"I would have put a two-way mirror on the bathroom door so I could have watched him. Maybe that way I would have had some privacy in the bathroom."

"Now that I have a child, looking back I wouldn't have spent so much time on fertility treatments and would have adopted a whole lot sooner. Or at least started the adoption process while I was trying to get pregnant just to cover all bases."

"If I had known then what I know now, I never would have gone back to work so quickly. I would have taken at least two years off. I felt a terrible rip every time I had to get ready for work and leave him with the babysitter. I still do. So, this year I am going to work only part time to make up for time lost."

"I would have started earlier, so that I could have had more than one child."

"I'm sorry I didn't have a rocking chair when she was an infant. I would have definitely spent the money on a rocking chair."

Resources

There are a *lot* of resources for mothers (midlife and otherwise) these days. Here are some highlights:

General Resources

Many online sites exist to help parents. Most have specialized areas where you can zone in on a topic or meet kindred spirits. Start here:

BabyZone.com (*www.babyzone.com*)
Large online neighborhood of resources for women pre-pregnancy through delivery and their kids zero to three years old. Check out the weekly "VIParent Newsletter" where—along with many other excellent articles—you will find my column, "Parenting in a Nutshell."

www.midlifemommies.com:
Connect with other mothers beyond thirty-five and over forty, link to places of specific interest, post on the message board and read other women's stories.

Mothers Who Think at *www.salon.com.* A site dedicated to keeping your mommy-brain intellectually challenged.

National Partnership for Women and Families
1875 Connecticut Ave., NW, Suite 650
Washington, D.C. 20009
202-986-2600
www.nationalpartnership.org
News, policies, government resources affecting women and their families.

National Association of Mothers
www.motherscenter.org
1-800-645-3828
New mother support and real-life centers.

National Parent Information Network
University of Illinois at Urbana-Champaign
Children's Research Center
51 Getty Drive
Champaign, IL 61820-7469
217-333-1386; 800-583-4135

Amongst my favorite parenting books are the *What to Expect* series (by Arlene Eisenberg et al.), which take you literally moment-by-moment through pregnancy, infancy and the toddler years. After that, you are on your own to find your way through the plethora of parenting magazines and books that guide you through every phase and stage of your little (and then big) one's life.

In addition, almost every community has a regional parenting publication, generally produced monthly, that includes a calendar of family events held locally. These are invaluable resources to get you connected in your own neighborhood.

U.S. Government Consumer Catalogs
Low-cost informative booklets on all kinds of topics. For one, try "How to Make College Affordable."

Infertility

RESOLVE
1310 Broadway
Somerville, MA 02144-1731
617-623-1156
Helpline: 617-623-0252
This well-known and well-respected nonprofit group goes above and beyond to help women with fertility and/or adoption concerns.

Adoption

National Adoption Information Clearinghouse
330 C Street, NW
Washington, D.C. 20447
888-251-0075
www.calib.com/naic

Adopt International
www.adoption.com/international
If you are adopting internationally, this is a good place to start.

Adoptive Families Magazine
P.O. Box 5159
Brentood, TN 37024
800-372-3300

AASK
657 Mission Street Suite 601
San Francisco, CA 94105
Adoption of Special Kids

An online search will turn up many agencies and facilitators. Some have photos of children who are waiting for families (i.e.: *www.adopt.org/adopt/* or *www.iaradopt.com*).

Aid to Adoption of Special Kids
501 E. Thomas Rd., Suite 100
Phoenix, AZ 85012
602-254-2275
800-370-2275
www.aask-az.org

Single Mothering

National Organization of Single Mothers
Box 68
Midland, NC 28107
www.singlemothers.org

Parents Without Partners
8807 Colesville Rd.
Silver Spring, MD 20910
800-637-7974
Chapters in each state.

Lesbian Mothering

Lesbian Mothers Support Society
P. O. Box 61, Station M
Calgary, Alberta, Canada T2P 269
403-265-6433
www.lesbian.org/lesbian-moms/
Legal, fertility and health issues.

Foster Mothering

National Foster Parent Association
www.nfpainc.org

Stay-at-Home Mothering

Mothers at Home
8310A Old Courthouse Road
Vienna, VA 22182
703-827-5903
www.mah.org.

Working

The Entrepreneurial Parent
Box 320722
Fairfield, CT 06432
http://en-parent.com
Resources for combining family and work.

National Association of Working Women's Job Survival
Hotline: 212-522-0925

"Everything a Working Mother Needs to Know" by Anne C.
Weisberg et al. A state-by-state summary of relevant legislation.

www.mothersandmore.com
For sequencing mothers (see the chapter on Working).

Pregnancy

Doulas of North America
1100 23rd Avenue
Seattle, WA 98112
206-324-5440
www.dona.com
AskDONA@aol.com

DONA Central Office
13513 N. Grove Dr.
Alpine, UT 84004
801-756-7331
1-800-311-BABY is a pregnancy hotline that links callers to state
    prenatal programs.

Surrogacy

Creating Families
1395 Bellaire Street
Denver, CO 80220
303-355-2107
www.eggdonor.net

Center for Surrogate Parenting, Inc.
Egg Donation, Inc.
West Coast office:
818-788-8288
East Coast office:
410-990-9860
www.creatingfamilies.com

Stepmothering

Stepfamily Association of America, Inc.
215 Centennial Mall South
Suite 212
Lincoln, NE 68508
800-735-0329
www.stepfam.org.

Childcare Referral

National Associationn of Child Care Resource
and Referral Agencies
1319 F St., NW
Suite 500
Washington, D.C. 20004-1106
202-393-5501
www.naccrra.net

Child Care Aware
800-424-2246
www.childcareaware.org